Arterial Grafting for Myocardial Revascularization

Indications, Surgical Techniques and Results

Ludwig K. von Segesser

With 127 Figures and 6 Tables

Springer-Verlag Berlin Heidelberg New York
London Paris Tokyo Hong Kong Barcelona

Ludwig K. von Segesser, M. D., F. A. C. S.
Clinic for Cardiovascular Surgery
Zürich University Hospital
CH-8091 Zürich, Switzerland

ISBN-13:978-3-642-75711-2 e-ISBN-13:978-3-642-75709-9
DOI: 10.1007/978-3-642-75709-9

Library of Congress Cataloging-in-Publication Data

Segesser, Ludwig K. von. Arterial grafting for myocardial revascularization : indications, surgical techniques, and results / Ludwig K. von Segesser.
Includes bibliographical references. Includes index.
ISBN-13:978-3-642-75711-2

1. Myocardial revascularization. 2. Internal thoracic artery–
– Transplantation. 3. Arterial grafts. I. Title.
[DNLM: 1. Coronary Artery Bypass. 2. Thoracic Arteries–transplantation. WG 169 S454a]
RD 598.35.M95S44 1990
617.4′12– –dc20
DNLM/DLC
for Library of Congress 90-10302 CIP

2124/3335-543210 – Printed on acid-free paper

Foreword

Cardiovascular disease, the leading cause of death in industrialized societies, not only strikes down a significant fraction of the population without warning, but also causes prolonged suffering and disability in even larger number. Until the development of heart surgery and the introduction of diagnostic techniques including cineangiography, stress electrocardiography, echocardiography, and myocardial scanning, the treatment of arteriosclerotic heart disease was confined to medical measures that were usually only partially effective.

After the introduction of selective coronary angiography by Sones, surgeons, led by Favaloro and Johnson, began to apply the principle of bypass to coronary arterial disease. Similar vascular techniques had already been developed for peripheral arterial occlusions in the femoral and popliteal vessels and employed the long saphenous vein as a conduit to extend pulsatile flow to the distal pedal arteries. The numbers of coronary bypass operations increased dramatically following the procedure's introduction.

Although the saphenous vein functioned very well, many patients were returning for reoperation between 5 and 10 years. Thus, the need for another bypass conduit became apparent. The internal mammary artery was the obvious choice. In 1964, Spencer first anastomosed an internal mammary artery to a large coronary artery. Four years later Green reported that he routinely used microsurgical techniques to bypass even smaller coronary vessels with the internal mammary artery. Others had expressed early interest in the mammary artery conduit, including Barner, Mills, and Loop. The mammary artery was used in most of these early series in selected patients and in selected arteries, in particular the left anterior descending artery.

With increased experience using the internal mammary artery, these groups of surgeons eventually applied the procedure to a larger population of patients. Eventually, the mammary artery was used in sequential fashion to bypass more than one artery, and, in some patients, both mammary arteries were used. Using these new techniques, surgeons could bypass almost every area of the diseased coronary system except the distal circumflex branches and distal right branches. Then, in 1983 and in 1985, Campeau and Lytle published the results of their long-term studies of mammary artery bypass. These important reports showed significantly different results in favor of the internal mammary artery over the saphenous vein graft. As a consequence of these studies, more surgeons reconsidered use of the internal mammary artery for the bypass conduit.

During the early period of coronary artery bypass surgery at the Texas Heart Institute, we usually reserved the mammary artery conduit for grafting to the left anterior descending coronary artery in younger patients, or for whenever the saphenous vein was not available. Because we believed in complete revascularization and treated many patients who were older and many who had diffuse disease, our use of the mammary graft was limited. As the technique used to perform mammary bypass changed over the years, however, to allow more complete revascularization, we began to use the internal mammary artery whenever possible.

Thus, the internal mammary progressed from the "no-conduit" days of internal mammary ligation of the 1930s to the indirect conduit of the 1960s; to the direct conduit of the 1970s; and to the double mammary, with or without sequential grafting in the 1980s. There is no question that in the 1990s complete revascularization using a proper combination of one or two mammary artery grafts, in addition to saphenous vein grafts appropriately placed to major vessels and their branches, is the state of the art in elective coronary artery surgery.

Surgeons as well as cardiologists have been impressed by the superior results that arterial conduits have over veins for bypass procedures. Consequently, they have looked elsewhere in the human anatomy for other sources of nonessential arteries. Early in the coronary bypass experience, the radial artery as a free graft was used, but curiously that artery seemed to be susceptible to atherosclerotic change. More recently, two arteries from the truncal anatomy (namely, the right gastroepiploic artery and the inferior epigastric artery) have been used with promising results. Meanwhile, surgeons will continue their enthusiastic use of the internal mammary artery because of its proven success and its convenient anatomic location near the heart.

To use the internal mammary artery well, however, we must understand its function and its indications. Ludwig von Segesser has carefully and studiously compiled all of the information we need to know about the internal mammary artery. Arterial Grafting for Myocardial Revascularization is a comprehensive contribution – from history, anatomy, and pathology to experimental and clinical studies, from clinical application to results, from complications to long-term follow-up – and will be a reference of inestimable value both to cardiologists and cardiovascular surgeons as they meet the needs of patients with coronary artery disease.

Denton A. Cooley, M. D.
Surgeon-in-Chief
Texas Heart Institute
Houston, Texas

Contents

Preface

πάντα ῥεῖ
perpetual flux

Heraktitos from Ephessos
550–480 B.C.

The importance of the internal mammary artery in treatment of coronary artery disease has changed over the years. This is illustrated not only by the fact that this vessel was renamed the internal thoracic artery but also by periods during which it was ligated with the idea of improving the coronary artery blood flow. Later on, the internal mammary artery was implanted into the myocardium and microvascular anastomoses were documented. However, the new blood flow brought to the myocardium was too limited to be effective. Since the introduction of coronary artery bypass grafting in the treatment of coronary artery disease in 1967, coronary artery revascularization has become the fastest growing form of surgery. Over many years, reversed saphenous veins were the preferred graft material for coronary artery revascularization. In the meanwhile, however, higher long-term patency rates have been achieved with internal mammary artery grafts than with saphenous vein grafts. These observations led to an exponential increase in the use of the internal mammary artery for coronary artery revascularization and the emergence of a number of new techniques, increasing its versatility. However, there have also been some negative experiences with this graft. The various experimental and clinical studies now available provide a growing basis for a scientific approach in internal mammary artery grafting.

The idea was for this book to relate my personal experience with the current state of knowledge as reported in the literature and to develop a philosophy of optimized internal mammary artery grafting for coronary artery revascularization.

For this purpose, I have analyzed many studies on the internal mammary artery – dealing with anatomy, pathology, experimental behavior in vitro and in vivo – and clinical reports. I have also established guidelines for internal mammary artery grafting that include indications, contraindications, surgical techniques, and steps for preventing or treating complications.

I wish to thank my teachers in surgery, B. Vogt (Lucerne), M. Allgöwer (Basel), A. Rohner (Geneva), R. Mégevand (Geneva), B. Faidutti (Geneva), D. A. Cooley (Houston), and M. Turina (Zürich), and all of my colleagues for the encouragement and assistance they have given me in my clinical work and writing.

I am grateful to M. Hegetschweiler, C. de Simio, O. Reinhard, and S. Wehrli for preparing artwork, and to the Experimental Surgical and Photoillustration Units of the Department of Surgery at Zürich University Hospital for their help. Finally, my thanks go to Springer-Verlag and its staff for the outstanding work in the production of this book.

Zürich, January 1990
Ludwig K. von Segesser

1 Introduction

Diseases of the cardiovascular system were responsible for 39.1% of all deaths registered during 1986 in Switzerland (range over the last 25 years: 39%–44%) as reported by the *Bundesamt für Statistik* and dominated all other causes such as malignant tumors (24.9%), accidents (8.3%), diseases of the respiratory system (6.7%), diseases of the nervous system (6.4%), metabolic disorders (3.9%), diseases of the digestive system (3.3%), and others (7.4%). As in other countries of the western hemisphere the diseases of the cardiovascular system were also the most frequent cause of hospitalization (21.9%), consultation of a medical doctor (14.8%), and prescription of an ambulatory treatment (17.6%) (Pharma Information 1988). Apart from the obviously severe consequences of cardiovascular diseases for the individual (morbidity and mortality), there can be no doubt about the micro- and macroeconomic impact of these diseases. This might explain the extremely rapid expansion in treatment of a single segment of cardiovascular diseases, that is coronary artery disease.

The construction of aortocoronary bypass grafts with reversed saphenous vein was introduced by Favaloro in 1967 (Favaloro et al. 1968 b). This procedure has been recognized as one of the most significant surgical advances ever. According to Loop et al. (1981) all operations performed in the United States from 1970 through 1978 increased approximately 25%. In contrast, coronary artery operations increased nearly 700% during those years. An estimated 180000 coronary artery operations are performed annually in the United States (Lefrak 1987).

Coronary artery bypass surgery improves the blood supply to territories supplied by blocked or narrowed arteries and it is generally agreed to be highly effective (Takaro et al. 1976; Kennedy et al. 1980; National Heart Lung and Blood Institute 1981; Loop 1981; European Coronary Surgery Study Group 1982; Braunwald et al. 1983; Turina 1987). Percutaneous transluminal angioplasty is another direct approach for limited coronary artery lesions (Grüntzig et al. 1979; Meier et al. 1985; Finci et al. 1987 a) as well as thrombolysis. Pure medical treatment, however, reduces angina by increasing the efficiency of the heart and reducing demand but it is much less sucessful than surgery in relieving symptoms and does little to improve the defective blood supply.

Surgical advances include improved myocardial protection and better perioperative care, which have resulted in a decrease in perioperative morbidity and mortality on one hand, and increasing technical skills, resulting from experience and expanded use of the internal mammary arteries, leading to improved long term results on the other.

2 Myocardial Revascularization and the Internal Mammary Artery

2.1 History of Myocardial Revascularization

The first approach for treatment of coronary artery disease was through the sympathetic nervous system. As early as 1899, Francois-Franck in France suggested a sympathectomy to relieve the pain of angina pectoris. Jonnesco (1920) performed a cervical thoracic ganglionectomy in 1916 as the first planned surgical attack on coronary artery disease, with the idea of increasing the blood flow to the heart by coronary artery vasodilatation. This however did not prove to be effective (McEachern et al. 1940) and the major role of cardiac denervation is relief of anginal pain. Other methods of cardiac denervation have been suggested such as pericoronary neurectomy (Fauteux and Swensen 1946), section of the preaortic plexus (Arnulf 1948), posterior rhizotomy (White 1955), and paravertebral nerve block (Mandl 1925). The disadvantage of these procedures, most of them with considerable surgical risk, remains the fact that they do not attack the basic coronary obstructive process. Different indirect approaches for reduction of angina pectoris such as surgical or medical ^{131}I thyroidectomy to reduce cardiac workload (Boas 1926; Blumgart et al. 1933) and carotid sinus nerve stimulation to reduce the heart's energy consumption (Braunwald et al. 1967) were also attempted.

Operations designed to augment the existing coronary blood supply are numerous. The fact that vascular anastomoses exist between the coronary circulation and the mediastinal circulation encouraged Beck in 1935 to produce vascular adhesions between the pericardium and the myocardium creating thereby a new source of blood to the surface of the heart. Other efforts for stimulation of collateral blood channels have included physical and chemical removal of the epicardium and the instillation of irritant or inflammatory materials such as talcum powder, sand, asbestos, phenol, hypertonic sodium salicylate, and Ivalon sponge. However the quantity of blood flow available has not proven significant. In order to bring larger quantities of blood into the myocardium, various grafts, such as pectoral muscle, stomach, liver, spleen, mediastinal fat, omentum with its vascular pedicle intact or as free graft, skin tubes, lung, and small intestine have been employed either, isolated or combined with de-epicardialization. All of them have been abandoned in favor of myocardial revascularization, even though some (pectoral muscle, omentum) are still used today for treatment of complicated wound healing disturbances after direct coronary artery revascularization.

Following the suggestion of Fieschi, ligation of both internal mammary arteries was performed to increase blood flow to the heart via the pericardiophrenic branches proximal to the ligatures, but subsequent double-blind studies failed to support the validity of this procedure (Cobb et al. 1959) and it has been abandoned.

Operations that produce coronary venous stasis or reversal of coronary circulation were advocated by Beck (1935) and referred to as Beck I (cardiopericardiopexy and stenosis of the coronary sinus between the posterior and middle cardiac veins) and Beck II (stenosis of the coronary sinus and reversal of flow through the coronary sinus by arterialization) operations. Only a few of the latter operations were performed because of the high associated mortality rate.

Augmentation of blood flow to the ischemic myocardium by grafting the internal mammary artery was begun by Vineberg in Montreal in 1945. He believed that if the internal mammary artery could be grafted successfully into the hypertrophied arteriolar collateral bed, which he knew to be characteristic of ischemic myocardium, blood flow to the myocardium would be augmented. Vineberg first published his concept in 1946 and began clinical application of his operation in 1950. However, the new blood flow brought to the myocardium appeared to be too limited to be effective as confirmed later (Beecher 1961; Wakabayashi et al. 1968; Yokoyama et al. 1972; Takara et al. 1985).

In 1954, Murray et al. reported a direct surgical approach with their experimental studies on anastomosis of the internal mammary artery to a coronary artery. Shortly thereafter, Longmire et al. (1958) in Los Angeles reported a series of patients in whom direct-vision coronary endarterectomy was carried out without cardiopulmonary bypass. Then Senning in Zürich (1961) reported patch grafting of a stenotic coronary artery with cardiopulmonary bypass.

The development of coronary cinearteriography by Sones at the Cleveland Clinic in the early 1960s (Sones and Shirey 1962) made possible the direct identification of stenotic and obstructive arteriosclerotic lesions in the coronary arteries and laid the groundwork for direct coronary artery revascularization.

In May 1967, Favaloro and Effler, at the Cleveland Clinic, began performing reversed saphenous vein grafting and in 1968 this technique was also applied by Hahn in Geneva (Hahn 1983). Favaloro, at that time in Buenos Aires, described the technique of the operation from the Cleveland Clinic (Favaloro 1968 b). Even earlier Garrett (1964), in Houston, successfully performed a reversed saphenous vein coronary artery bypass graft to the left anterior descending coronary artery in an unplanned way (Garrett et al. 1973).

In the meantime Spencer et al. (1964) described experimental internal mammary artery coronary artery grafting and Green et al. in New York performed, following experimental studies presented in 1965, the anastomosis of the distal end of the left internal mammary artery to the anterior descending coronary artery using the dissecting microscope clinically in February 1968.

Kolesov in Leningrad had already performed the first sutured internal mammary artery–coronary artery end-to-end anastomosis in a man with class III angina on 25 February 1964 (Kolesov and Potashov 1965; Kolesov 1967). However, his contributions to coronary artery revascularization were not recognized or appreciated at that time, even in his own country and only became known to a larger public by the reports of Effler et al. (1971), Spencer (1983), Tector (1986), and Olearchyk (1986, 1988).

In 1971 Flemma et al. described the technique of sequential grafting, in which one vein was used for several distal anastomoses. The advantages of this technique were further enhanced by the studies of Bartley et al. (1972) and Sewell (1974). The use of the right and left internal mammary arteries for direct revascularizations were reported by Suzuki in 1973 and by Barner in 1974 (Favaloro 1968a had already reported bilateral internal mammary artery implants). The first reports on patency rates after internal mammary coronary artery anastomoses appeared in 1974 (Kay et al. 1974) and 1976 (Barner et al. 1976).

In 1976 Siegel and Loop reported higher patency rates for internal mammary artery grafts in comparison to saphenous vein grafts for coronary artery revascularization and in 1977 Loop et al. identified the higher patency rate of internal mammary artery grafts as a factor responsible for improved survival. Singh (1983) found that the long-term performance of the internal mammary artery grafts is far superior to the saphenous vein grafts and Tector described the internal mammary artery as the best choice for bypass of the diseased left anterior descending coronary artery. In the same year Kabbani reported sequential internal mammary-coronary artery bypass.

In the late seventies the term "internal mammary artery" was officially changed to "internal thoracic artery". However, this modification did not have the expected impact and over 90% of the studies published since continue to use the term "internal mammary artery" for this vessel.

Superior 10 year results of internal mammary grafts compared to saphenous veins were reported by Grondin (1984), Okies et al. (1984), Loop et al. (1986 a), and Olearchyk and Magovern (1986), and superior 15 year results were published by Cameron et al. (1986). These observations led to an exponential increase in the use of the internal mammary artery, including isolated mammary anastomoses, sequential anastomoses (i.e. anastomosis of the mammary artery with more than one coronary artery), bilateral mammary anastomoses, and all sorts of combinations.

If patency rates and long-term results after coronary artery bypass are superior when the internal mammary artery, rather than the saphenous vein, is used as a bypass graft, as listed by 84% of 750 surveyed surgeons performing myocardial revascularization in the United States, it appears indeed surprising that only 30% of them use the internal mammary artery in at least 90% of their operations (Lefrak 1987).

2.2 Indications for Surgical Coronary Artery Revascularization Today

Surgical coronary artery revascularization has been an established means of treatment of coronary artery disease since the early 1970s. The big randomized studies (National Heart, Lung and Blood Institute 1981; European Coronary Surgery Study Group 1982; Takaro et al. 1976; CASS Principal Investigators et al. 1983; Alderman et al. 1983; Veterans Administration Coronary Artery Bypass Surgery Cooperative Study Group 1984; Passamini et al. 1985; Varnauskas et al. 1988; Killip 1988) have not only shown the effectiveness of coronary artery surgery in respect to relief of angina, but also in respect to prolongation of life. This was despite the limitations of these analyses, e.g., the fact that patients assigned to the medical group undergoing surgical revascularization during the follow-up period remained in the medical group for analyses of the outcome. On the other hand important therapeutic tools available today, such as percutaneous coronary artery angioplasty, were not available at the time of randomization for these studies. A considerable part of previously surgical patients with one- or two-vessel disease are nowadays treated by the invasive cardiologist with angioplasty, thrombolysis, and recanalization. Surgical coronary artery revascularization is now mainly indicated in patients in whom the invasive cardiologist was not successful or in whom the disease is judged too advanced for nonsurgical revascularization.

Accepted indications for therapeutic surgical coronary artery revascularization include:

- stable angina in patients with multivessel disease and a left ventricular ejection fraction of more than 20%
- unstable angina in patients with failed or contraindicated percutaneous transluminal angioplasty
- residual coronary artery stenosis after thrombolysis in acute myocardial infarction
- persistent angina after myocardial infarction

Prophylactic coronary artery bypass surgery in the presence of documented ischemia appears to be indicated in oligo- and asymptomatic patients with:

- significant stenosis of the left main coronary artery
- severe three-vessel disease
- significant proximal stenoses of the left anterior descending coronary artery and circumflex coronary artery
- significant coronary artery disease and major abdominal or thoracic surgery as well as other cardiac surgery (valves, congenital heart disease)

From the surgeon's point of view, however, the criteria for evaluation of surgical treatment in coronary artery disease have moved over the last few years from the standard classification into one-, two-, and three-vessel disease and quality of left ventricular ejection fraction to the quantity of myocardial mass at risk of ischemia (infarction) and long-term bypass patency rates.

Because of the increased risk of perioperative morbidity and mortality in reoperations for coronary artery disease relative to primary operations (Lytle et al. 1987) the former appear to be indicated mainly for patients with severe clinical impairment (Egloff et al. 1984). In patients with severely impaired myocardial function (left ventricular ejection fraction below 20%), other forms of treatment such as heart transplantation (von Segesser et al. 1989) and possibly mechanical circulatory support (von Segesser et al. 1988a) have to be considered.

2.3 Early and Late Results of Coronary Artery Bypass Grafting: Attrition of Saphenous Vein Grafts

The early mortality of coronary artery bypass grafting showed a progressive decrease from the early 1970s when it reached up to 12% (Robinson 1978). In the current era mortality approaches zero (Kirklin et al. 1986). This evolution can also be documented for Zürich as shown by Lioupis (1988). With this progress coronary artery bypass grafting also became available for elderly patients (Elayda et al. 1984) and combined with other cardiac and noncardiac surgical procedures (Cooley et al. 1978), as well as in patients with a variety of serious coexisting medical problems, such as renal failure (Love et al. 1980), coagulopathies (Dorros et al. 1981) and pregnancy (Majdam et al. 1983).

Despite the growing success of coronary artery bypass surgery (performed by 95% of surgeons exclusively with saphenous vein grafts), increasing evidence of progressive attrition of the saphenous vein grafts appeared. Although more attention was paid to saphenous vein graft preparation, complete revascularization was advocated, use of antiplatelet drugs was introduced, control of coronary artery spasm was improved, and angioplasty of vein grafts, graft anastomoses, and distal coronary arteries became available the number of reports on saphenous vein bypass occlusion (Frey et al. 1984), redo coronary artery bypass procedures (Loop et al. 1976) and the superiority of the internal mammary artery as graft material (Singh et al. 1983, Grondin 1984, Okies et al. 1984) increased (see also Sects. 8.3 and 10.3).

In a series of 250 consecutive coronary artery revascularization procedures performed with saphenous vein grafts in the late 1970s there were 14 reinterventions (5.6%) (Faidutti and von Segesser 1985). The interval between first and second operation was less than 1 year in one case (early reoperation) and more than 1 year (late reoperation) in 13 cases: mean 5.9 years (range 2–10 years). Similar intervals are reported in the literature (Cosgrove et al. 1986, Lytle et al. 1987) and reflect the reduced patency rate of only 50% of saphenous vein grafts implanted onto the left anterior descending coronary artery after 7.5 years as reported by Lytle et al. (1983) and others.

Two types of mechanism can be observed in patients with venous aortocoronary artery bypass failure:

- early thrombosis suggesting a technical problem or inadequate runoff (bypass thrombosis without macroscopic lesions of the bypass wall)
- late thrombosis, suggesting progression of the arterial lesions, attrition of the bypass itself or both.

Changes in the native vessels following aortocoronary bypass operation were analyzed by Goebel et al. (1983) in a prospective study of 238 men 3 months after coronary artery revascularization and 5 months after preoperative angiography. Progression was defined as increase of stenosis of at least 20% or new total occlusion. Progression was significantly more frequent in vessels with than without bypass and was located proximally to the anastomosis in most cases, less frequently at the anastomosis, and very rarely distally to the anastomosis. Proximal progression was significantly more frequent with patent than with occluded bypasses. Stenoses at the anastomoses were significantly more frequent with occluded than

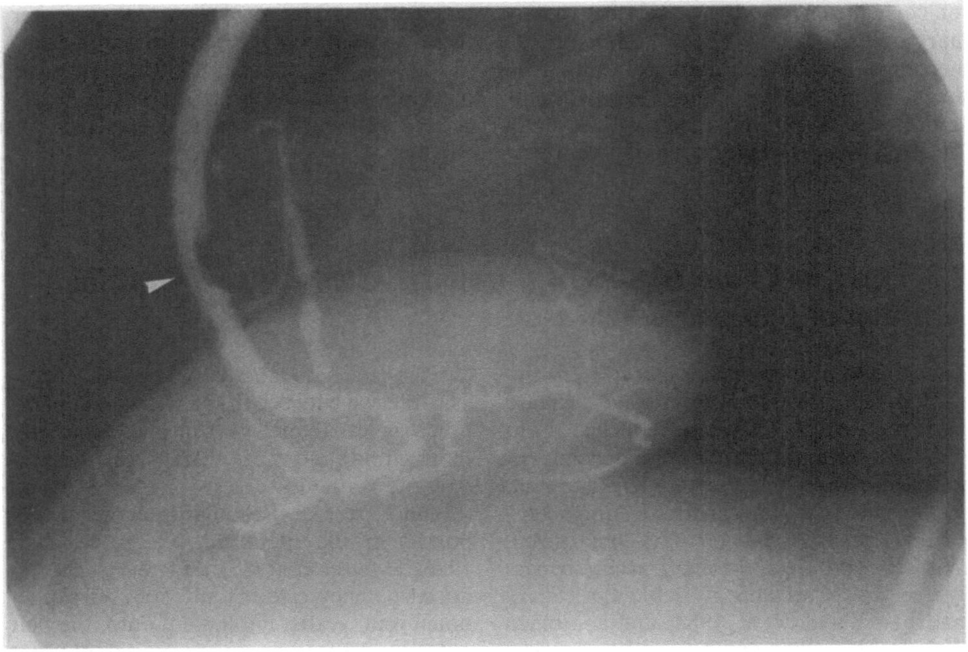

Fig. 1. Coronary angiogram showing saphenous vein graft implanted onto the distal right coronary artery 4 years earlier with significant stenosis (*arrow*) due to atheromatous bypass attrition.

Fig 2. Coronary angiogram showing a severe lesion (*arrow*) of a saphenous vein bypass graft implanted onto the left anterior descending coronary artery 6 years earlier

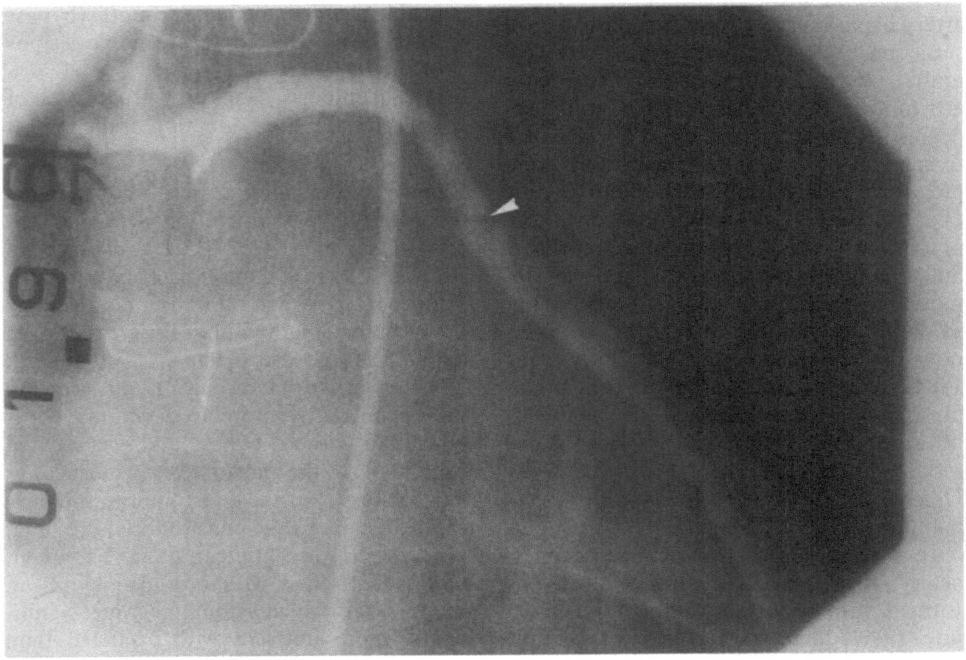

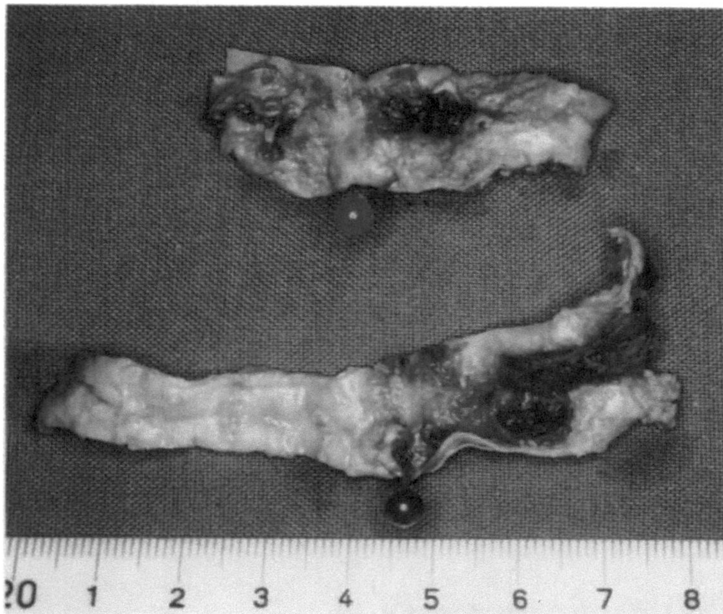

Fig. 3. Macroscopic view of an opened saphenous vein graft explanted after 6 years (same case as Fig. 2): exulcerated atheromatous lesion (*upper graft*) and atheromatous graft lesions with partial thrombosis (*lower graft*)

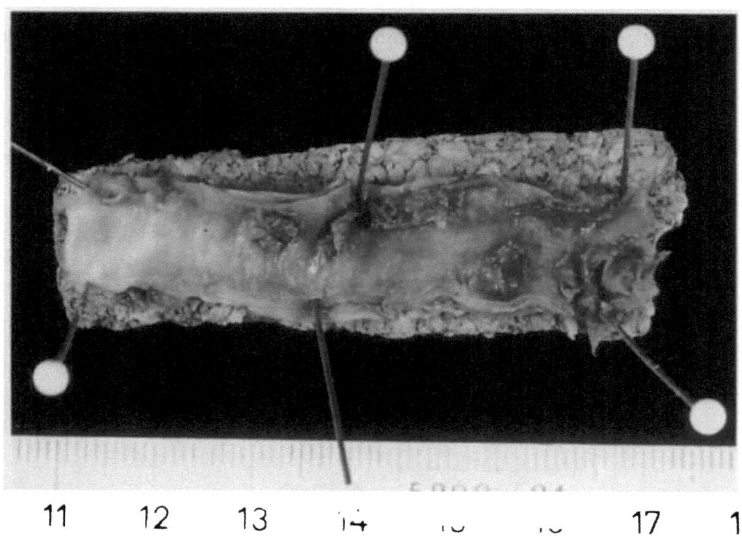

Fig 4. Macroscopic view of a saphenous vein graft with severe atheromatous attrition explanted after 5 years

with patent bypasses. Stenoses of a higher degree had a stronger tendency for progression than slighter stenoses. Regression was rare and nearly always caused by surgery (endarterectomy).

Various lesions of the bypass itself or its wall can be observed. Intimal hyperplasia can occur in the early postoperative period. Later on there are stenoses (Figs. 1, 2) and ulcerations can occur (Fig. 3) as a result of atherosclerotic disease (Figs. 4–6) of the venous graft on one hand and aneurysms of the graft on the other. The latter can be segmentary, at the level of a former valve (Fig. 7) or all over the graft. In some cases these lesions occur very early (after a few months) and in others their development needs years.

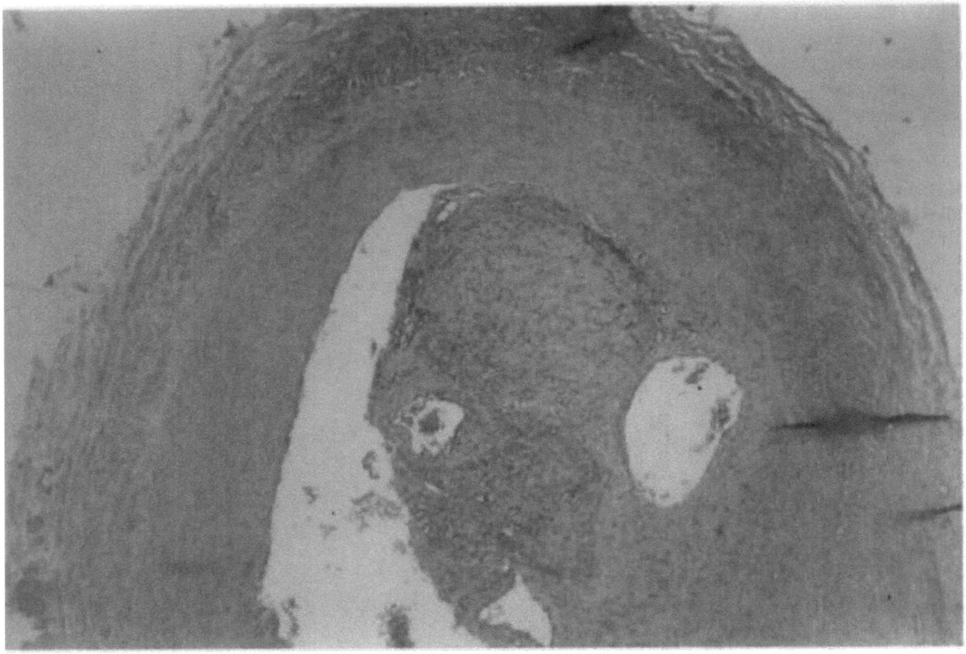

Fig. 5. Microscopic view of a thrombosis due to atheromatosis in a saphenous vein graft removed 5 years after implantation (same case as Fig. 4). H & E, ×10

Fig. 6. Microscopic view of a thrombosed saphenous vein graft (same case as Figs. 4 and 5) with important intimal thickening. van Gieson, ×20

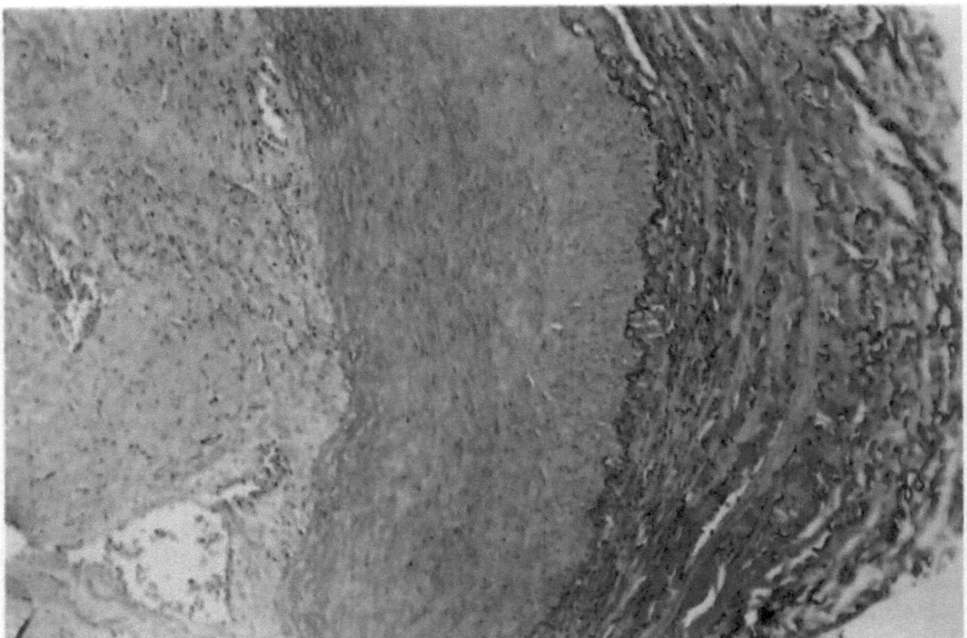

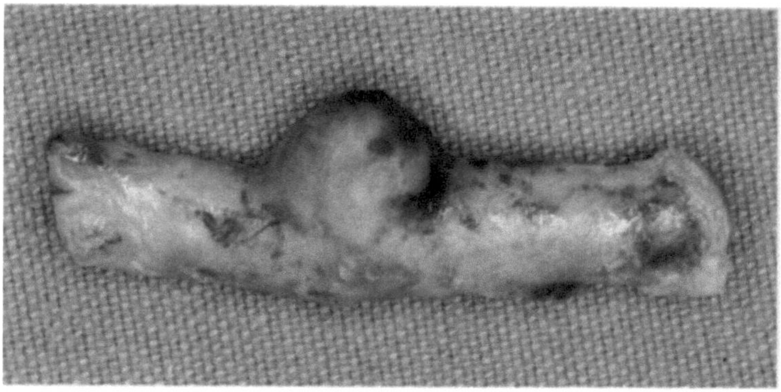

Fig. 7. Segmental aneurysmal dilatation of a thrombosed saphenous vein graft removed after 8 years at redo coronary artery revascularization.

The occurrence of early graft thrombosis (during the first year) due to platelet deposition can be reduced with platelet inhibitor therapy as reported by Chesebro et al. (1984) and Fuster and Chesebro (1986). However, the best way to avoid early and late saphenous vein graft failure in aortocoronary bypass grafting is to avoid using the saphenous vein as graft material and to use systematically the internal mammary arteries (Killip 1988) for the coronary artery revascularization procedures.

3 Anatomy of the Internal Mammary Artery

3.1 Normal Anatomy

3.1.1 Macroscopic Studies

The internal mammary artery is a very constant vessel, which can be found paramedial, on the right and left anterior, inner thoracic wall. It should therefore be termed more correctly the internal thoracic artery (see also Sect. 2.1). However, it has entered the literature as the internal mammary artery and is cited as such in over 90% of the papers dealing with it.

The internal mammary artery (right and left) is an unusual artery in that it is fed from its proximal end by the subclavian artery, through its midportions it supplies arterial blood to the intercostal arteries, and it anastomoses distally to the iliac artery by the epigastric artery and to the aorta by the musculophrenic arteries.

The proximal origin of the internal mammary artery, either right or left, is on the concavity of the subclavian artery, just opposite to the thyrocervical trunk which is the second branch on the convexity of the subclavian artery (the first branch is the vertebral artery). After crossing the subclavian veins the internal mammary arteries line the sternum on both sides in a distance of about 1–2 cm from the sternal border. They are accompanied in general by one or two internal mammary veins which drain into the subclavian vein and some lymphatic vessels and lymph nodes.

After a proximal, medial thymic branch (Fig. 8), the internal mammary artery anastomoses with the intercostal arteries beyond each rib until it reaches the sixth intercostal space where it divides in two major branches. The craniocaudal branch enters the sheath of the musculus rectus abdominis and anastomoses with the superior epigastric artery whereas the major lateral branch follows the cartilaginous arch of the ribs. The internal mammary vessels which lie directly on the chondral part of the ribs are covered on the inner side by the musculus transversus thoracis, the strong inner thoracic fascia, and the pleura.

There is no major difference between the right and left internal mammary arteries, with one exception. In its proximal part the left internal mammary artery runs very close to the thoracic cage whereas on the right side, there can be up to 1 cm of connective tissue between the proximal part of the internal mammary artery and the ribs. This might be due to the different anatomy of the subclavian arteries which originate on the left side from the aorta and on the right side from the brachiocephalic trunk.

3.1.2 Microscopic Studies

Histological analyses have shown that the proximal part of the internal mammary artery has in general to be classified as elastic artery and the distal part as muscular artery. The microscopic view of a normal section of an internal mammary artery is given in Fig. 9. Landymore and Chapman (1987) have shown in an analysis of five internal mammary artery pedicles that the vasa vasorum were confined to the adventitia and did not penetrate the medial layer of the artery. The distance from the lumen to the outermost portion of the media measured 200 ± 67 µm (mean $\pm$ standard error of the mean: 1567 measurements). One internal mammary artery was studied in detail. The mean thickness of the endothelium and subendothelial collagen was 2.5 µm, the internal elastic lamina measured 180 µm. There were nine other elastic layers. The adventitia, which abutted on the surrounding fat, had a thickness of 100 µm and consisted of longitudinal collagen fibers and fine longitudinal elastin fibrils.

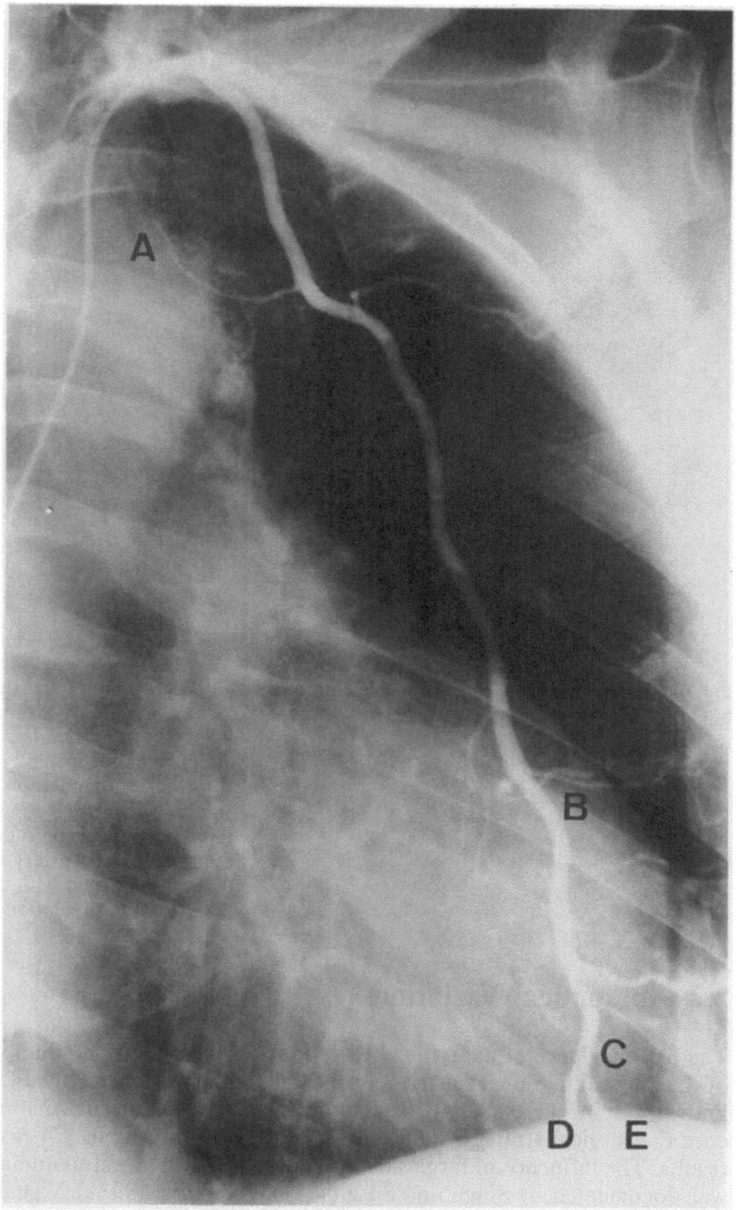

Fig. 8. Selective arteriography of the left internal mammary artery showing its origin from the left subclavian artery and the craniocaudal parasternal anatomical situation including:

A first medial thymic branch,
B anastomoses with the intercostal arteries
C distal bifurcation, with
D craniocaudal branch anastomosing with the superior epigastric artery, and
E lateral branch

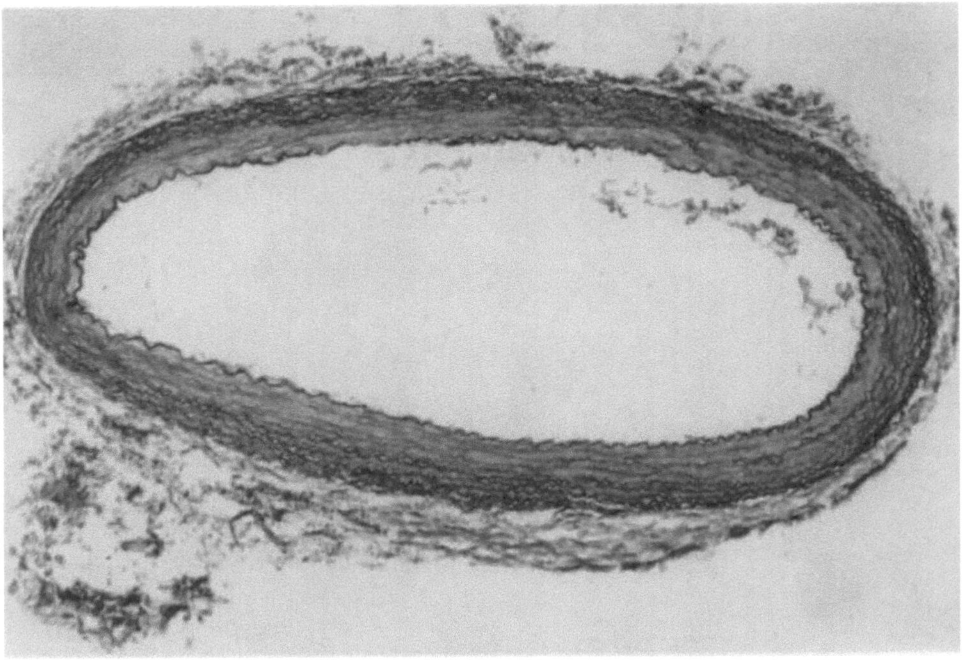

Fig. 9. Microscopic view of a normal section of a human internal mammary artery (no intimal thickening)

Fig. 10. Angiographic demonstration of the left ▷ internal mammary artery with:
A large side branch (50% of internal mammary artery in diameter),
B tortuosity (angulation > 90°)

Fig. 11. Angiographic demonstration of left in- ▷ ternal mammary artery showing:
A common origin with otherlarge branches,
B tortuosity (angulation > 90°)

3.2 Anatomical Variations

The true incidence of anatomical variations of the internal mammary arteries is not well known despite the fact that they can influence the surgical strategy and even surgical results. The influence of large side branches was documented by Singh and Sosa (1981), and Singh and Magovern (1982) and confirmed by Pelias and Del Rossi (1985).

In a serial study performed at Zürich University (Bauer et al. 1988), the internal mammary artery was visualized angiographically in 145 consecutive patients (39–82 years of age, mean 57.5) undergoing cardiac catheterization prior to cardiac surgery. Satisfactory visualization was possible in 249/290 internal mammary arteries studied (86%); it was better in left internal mammary arteries (140/145: 97%) than in right internal mammary arteries (109/145: 75%). In this series the left internal mammary artery was used for grafting in 124 cases (86%) whereas the right internal mammary artery was used in 57 cases (39%). Visualization of the internal mammary artery was free of complications in all patients. Early mortality of coronary artery bypass grafting in this series of elective surgery was 0%. A total of 60 surgically significant anomalies was observed in 44 patients (30%):

- large side branches defined as at least 50% of internal mammary artery diameter (Fig. 10): 24 cases (9.6% of analyzed internal mammary arteries)

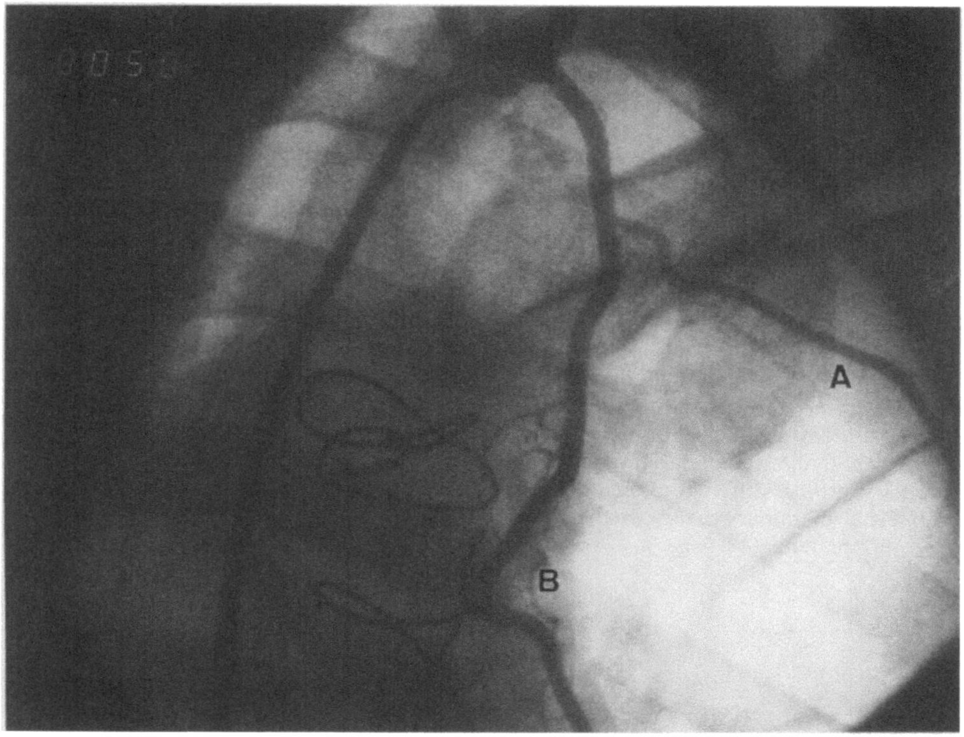
A
B

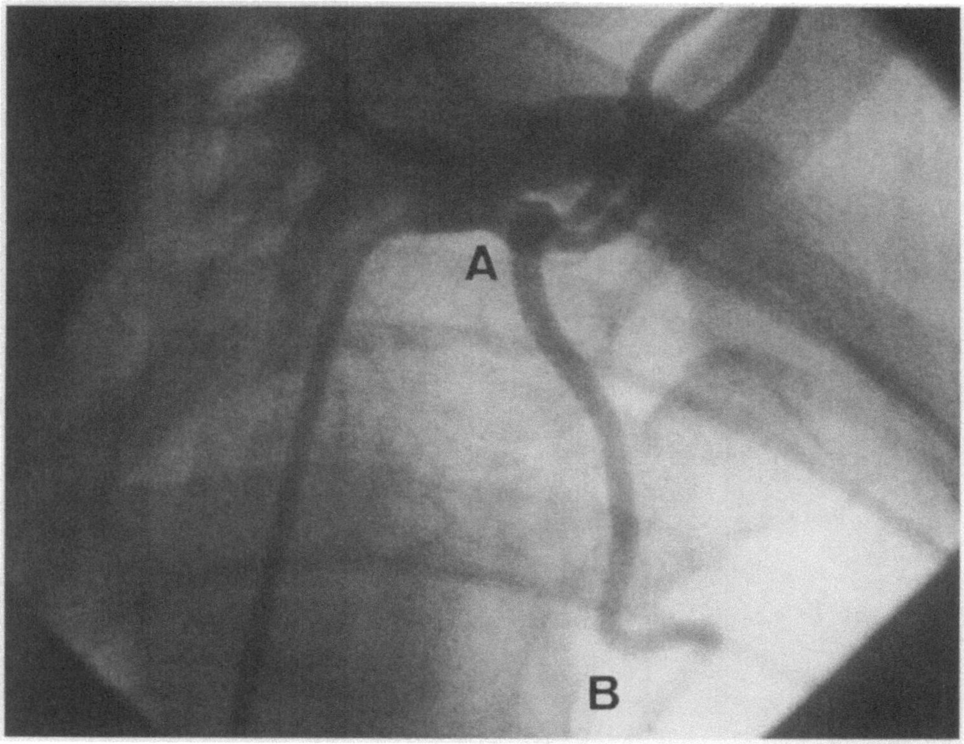
A
B

- common origin of the internal mammary artery with another major artery, (e.g., thyrocervical trunk, vertebral artery, or others: Fig. 11): 22 cases (8.8%)
- tortuosity defined as angulations of more than 90° (Figs. 10, 11): 9 cases (3.6%)
- atypical origin or course of the internal mammary artery (Fig. 12): 3 cases (1.2%)
- spastic reaction of the internal mammary artery: 1 case (0.4%)
- atheriosclerotic lesions of the internal mammary artery: 1 case (0.4%)

Angiographic visualization of the internal mammary artery resulted in modification of surgical strategy as ligation of major proximal branches, rejection of narrowed internal mammary artery, different preparation of the internal mammary artery in the upper chest, in 7 patients (4.8%).

This analysis shows that significant anomalies of the internal mammary arteries are not rare. In contrast to the opinion of Barner (1974b), we believe that some of them can escape during internal mammary artery take down and might, when unrecognized, jeopardize internal mammary artery flow after coronary bypass grafting. The case reported by Tartini et al. (1985) is a typical example of a variation of the internal mammary artery causing residual pain after internal mammary-coronary artery anastomosis.

Other anomalies such as the one reported by Robicsek et al. in 1967, where the anterior interventricular (descending) coronary artery and vein originate from the left internal mammary vessels, have also to be considered.

Fig. 12. Angiographic demonstration of left internal mammary artery with: A atypical lateral origin, B normal origin near vertebral artery

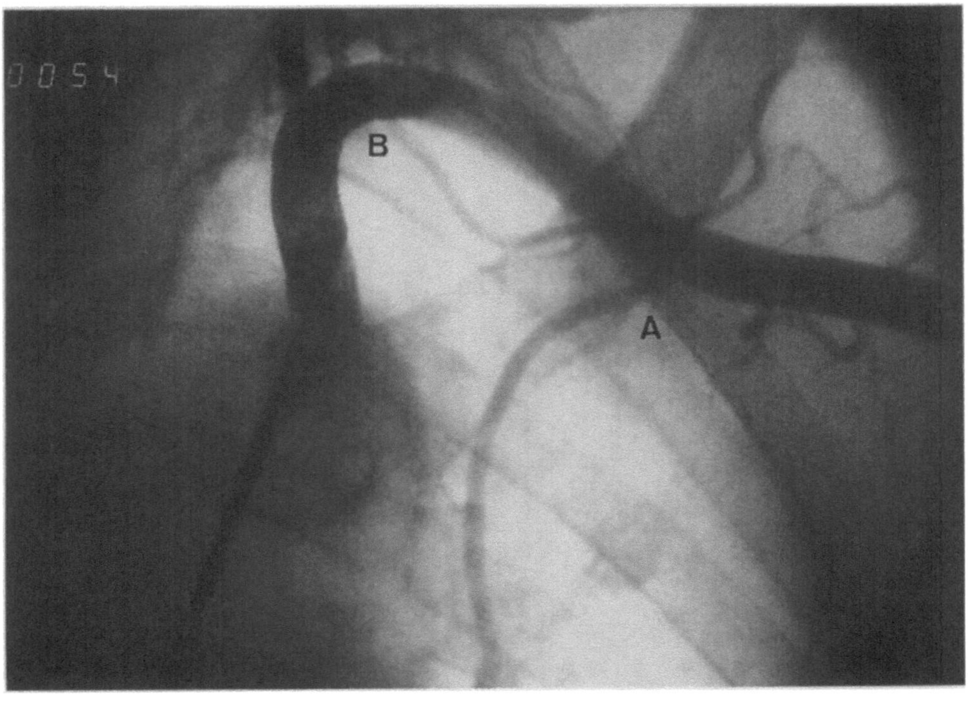

4 Pathology of the Internal Mammary Artery and the Subclavian Artery

4.1 Angiographic Studies

The internal mammary artery is known for a low incidence of pathologic lesions. However, the serial studies of Bauer et al. (1988) have shown not only that anatomical variations appear in a significant percentage, but also that pathologic lesions, such as atheromatous stenoses of the internal mammary artery (Fig. 13) and the subclavian artery (Fig. 14) can be documented by angiography. If stenosed internal mammary arteries are not used for coronary artery revascularization because of limited or absent additional flow, the subclavian artery stenoses can lead to additional symptoms due to coronary–subclavian steal as reported by Brown (1977), Tyras and Barner (1977) and Bashour et al. (1984). The internal mammary artery appears also to be useless in patients with aortic isthmus stenosis as macroscopic atheromatosis is visible in these dilated vessels (M. Turina, Zürich, personal communication).

Angiographic studies also allow one to distinguish between functional subclavian artery compression (Fig. 15) which is reversible (Fig. 16) and irreversible atheromatous lesions (Fig. 14). Fixed internal mammary artery stenoses (Fig. 13) can be distinguished from spastic reactions by injection of standard vasodilating agents used

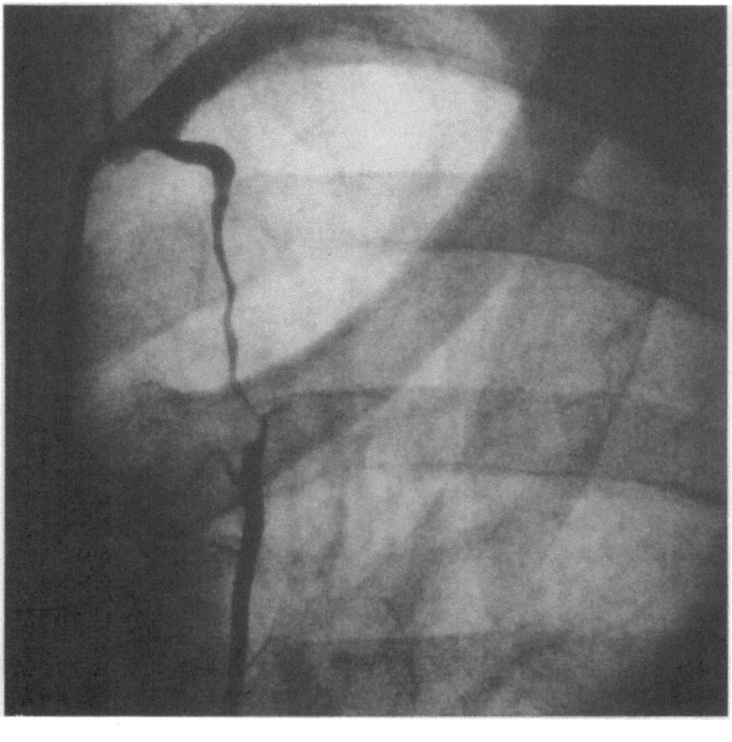

Fig. 13. Angiography of the left internal mammary artery showing moderate atheromatous plaque at the level of the subclavian artery and severe stenosis of the internal mammary artery

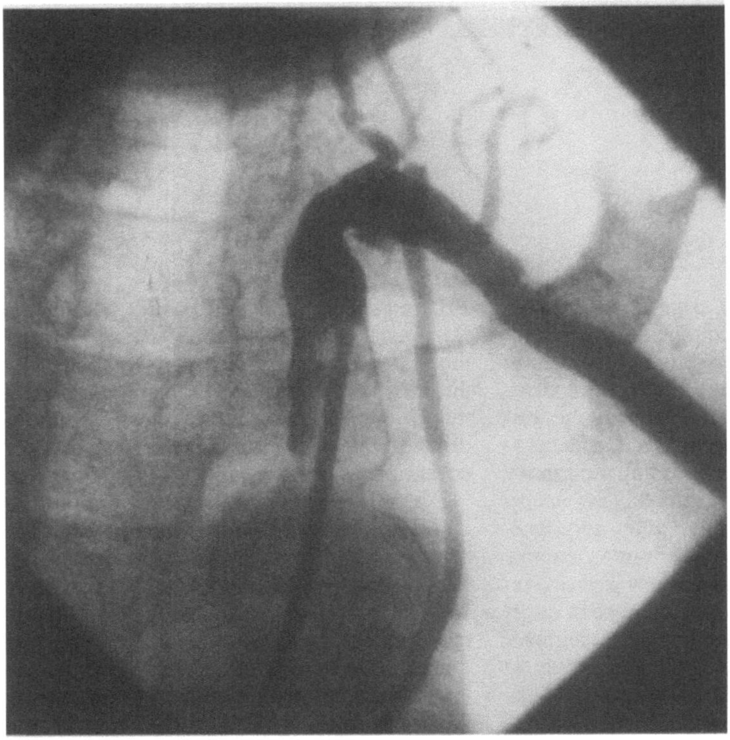

Fig. 14. Angiography of the left subclavian artery showing moderate stenosis of this vessel proximal to the origin of the internal mammary artery

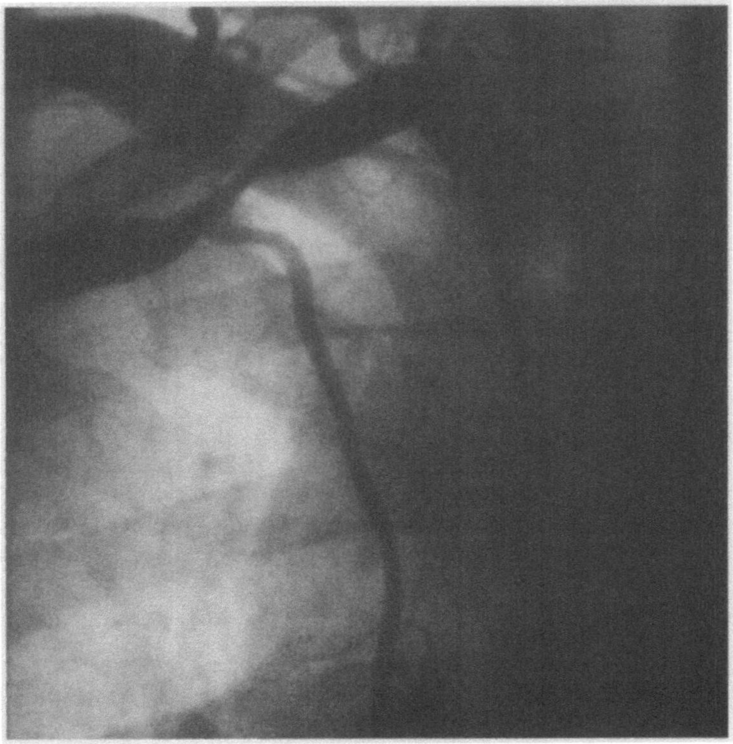

Fig. 15. Angiography of the right subclavian artery with important stenosis proximal to the internal mammary artery. This lesion is due to extrinsic compression as shown by Fig. 16 obtained from the same patient during the same catheterization procedure

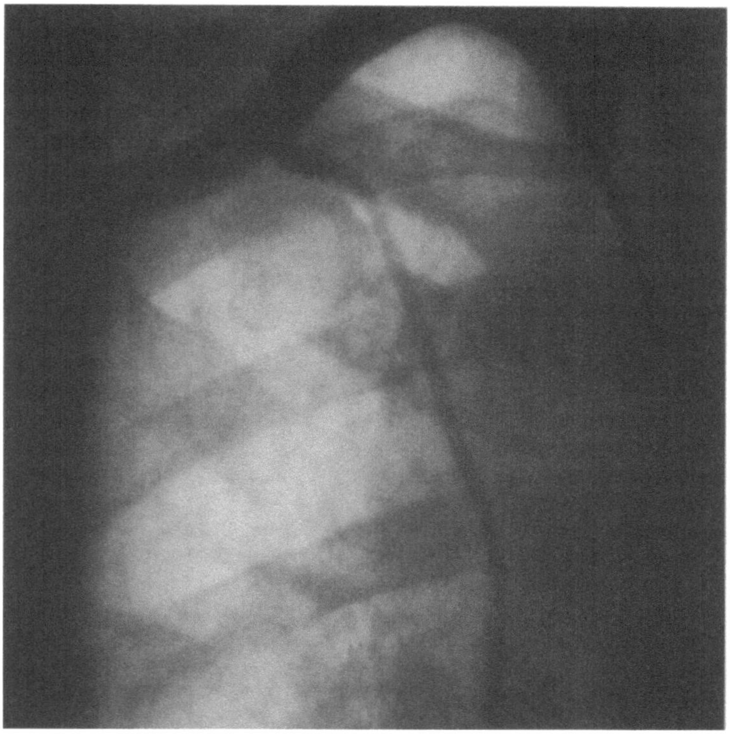

Fig. 16. Relief of the extrinsic stenosis of the subclavian artery achieved by adduction of the right upper extremity (same patient as Fig. 15)

Fig. 17. Angiographic demonstration of an arteriovenous fistula between the right internal mammary artery and the superior caval vein in a patient with aortic and mitral valve replacement 6 years earlier

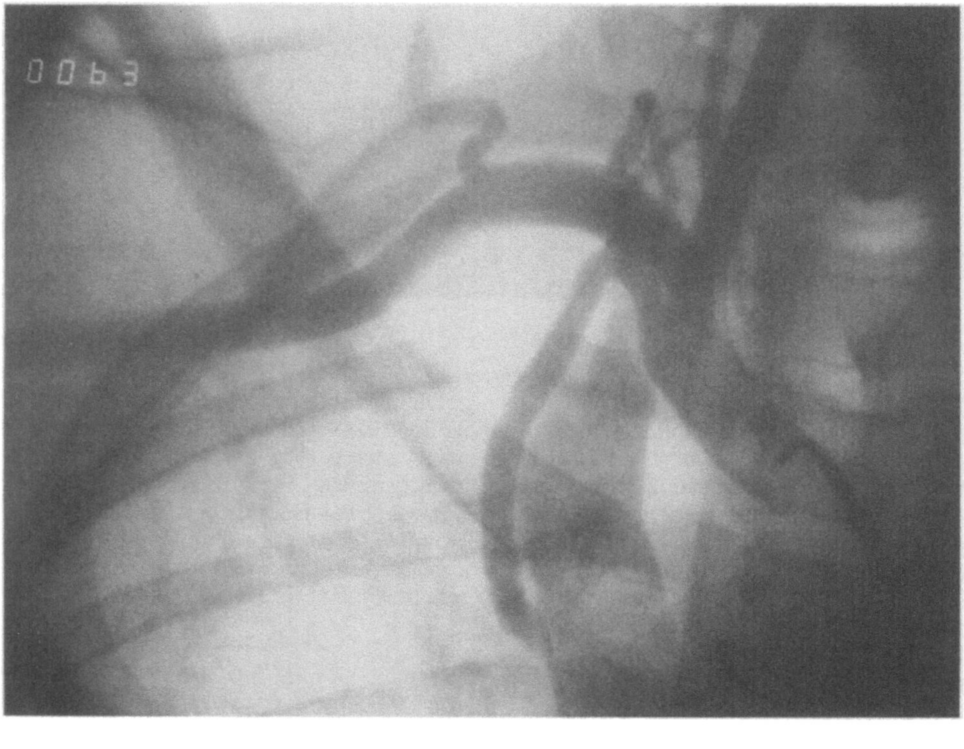

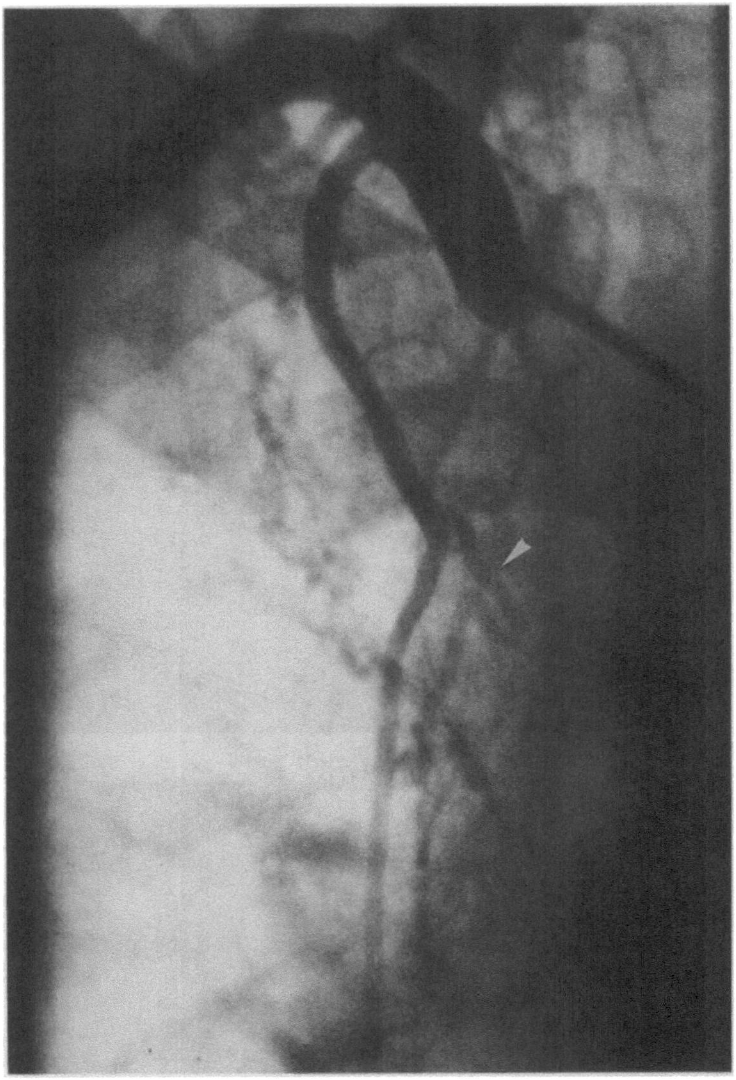

Fig. 18. Angiography of abnormal vessels in the region of the right internal mammary artery (unknown cause)

during coronary angiography. Other conditions, such as internal mammary artery to superior caval vein fistulas (Fig. 17) or abnormal vessels (Fig. 18) can also be demonstrated. Further pathological lesions such as aneurysm of the subclavion artery involving the origin of the internal mammary artery (Rainer et al.1973) and especially for redo procedures, internal mammary artery ligation by peristernal wires as well as internal mammary artery arteriovenous fistulas (Maher et al. 1982) have also been reported.

Digital subtraction angiography can also be used for screening of the internal mammary arteries (Fig. 19) as it allows one to identify absent (Fig. 20), hypoplastic or stenotic internal mammary arteries (Fig. 21). However, conventional angiography shows superior resolution and allows more accurate analysis (Fig. 22).

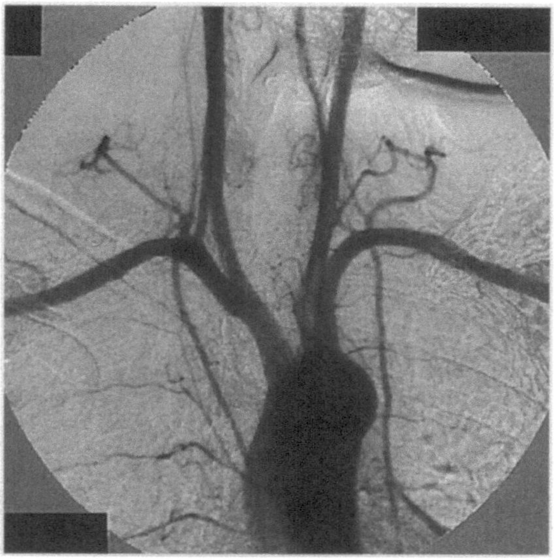

Fig. 19. Digital subtraction angiography of the aortic arch and the supra-aortic vessels with demonstration of patent right and left internal mammary arteries

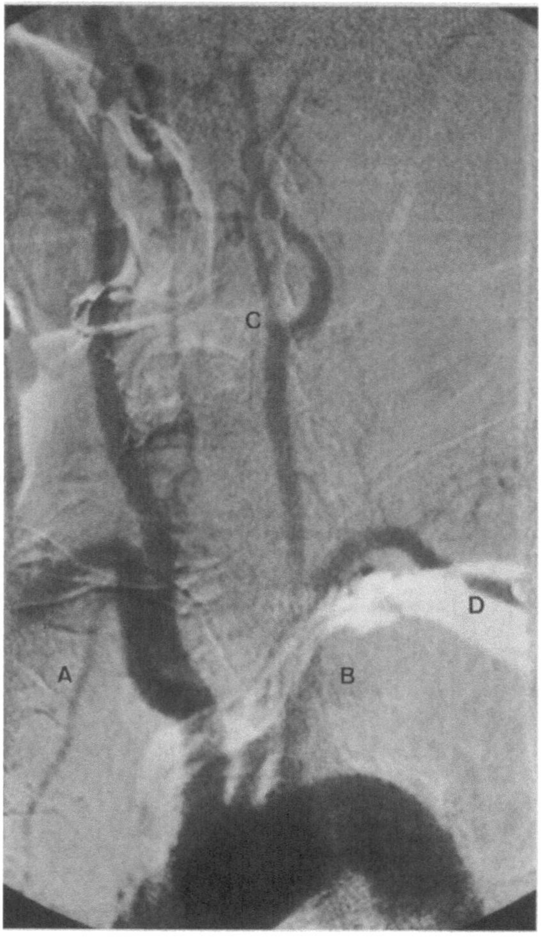

Fig. 20. Digital subtraction angiography of the aortic arch and supra-aortic vessels showing:

A right internal mammary artery,
B absent left internal mammary artery,
C left internal carotid artery stenosis, and
D left subclavian vein

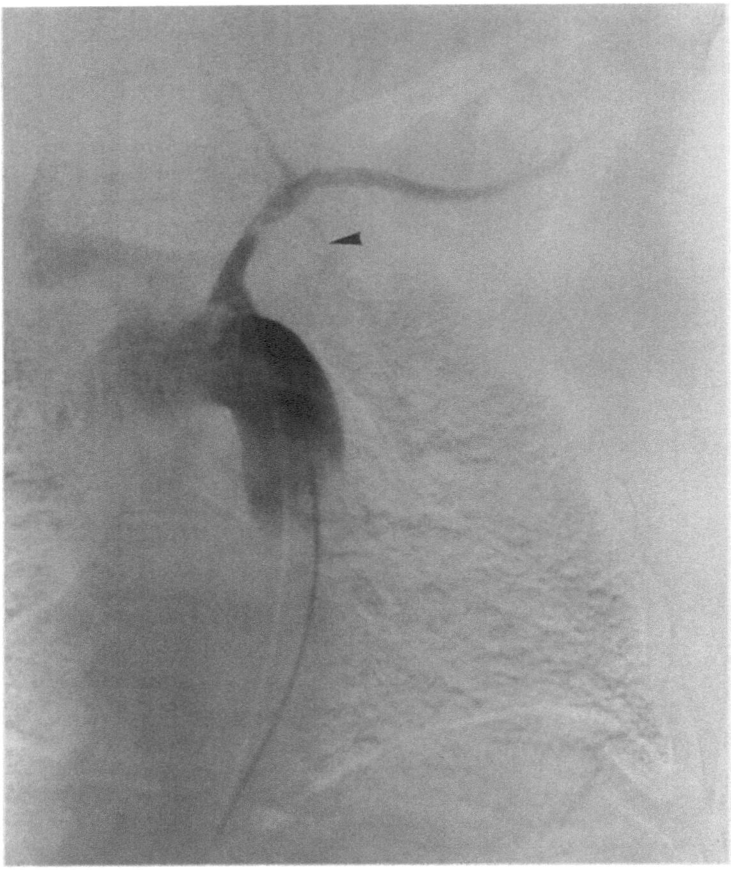

Fig. 21. Digital subtraction angiography showing hypoplastic left internal mammary artery

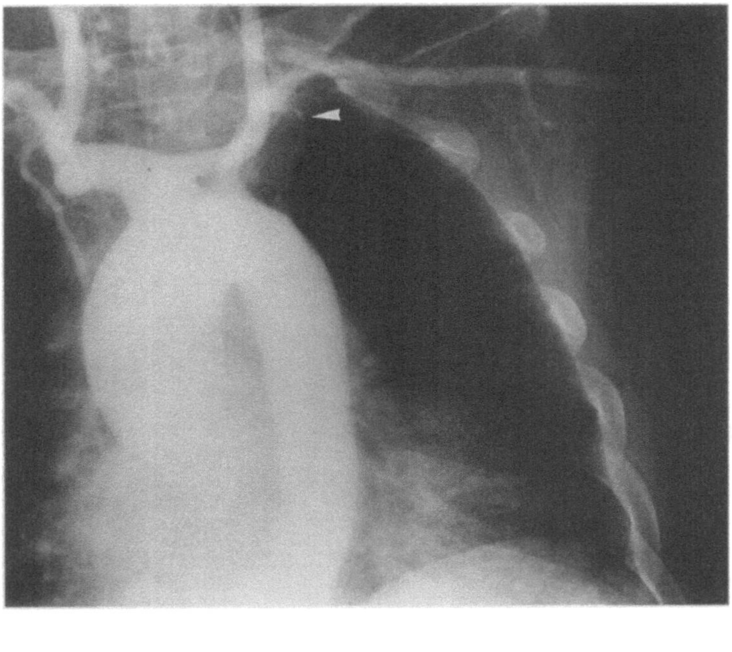

Fig. 22. Conventional angiography confirming hypoplasia of the left internal mammary artery (same case as Fig. 21)

4.2 Microscopic Studies

Despite the low incidence of pathologic lesions of the internal mammary artery (Lindenau et al. 1976, Nemes et al. 1977) there are some reports in the literature dealing with atherosclerosis of the internal mammary artery. In 1974 Frazier et al. reported three patients undergoing coronary artery bypass operation who were found to have significant atherosclerotic disease involving the internal mammary artery. Kay et al. (1976) evaluated the incidence of atherosclerosis in the internal mammary artery in 215 segments from routine postmortem examinations microscopically. Significant atherosclerotic narrowing was seen in nine patients (4.2%). No patient had more than 50% reduction in lumen diameter. The degree of incipient atherosclerosis correlated well with age, hypertension, diabetes and peripheral vascular disease. Mestres et al. (1986) analyzed 38 segments of the internal mammary artery obtained at the time of coronary artery surgery and 20 segments obtained at postmortem studies. Severe disease, with more than 50% luminal narrowing was found in one necropsy case (5%) and in no surgical case. Luminal reduction between 25% and 50% was found in one case of the surgical group. The remaining sections were normal or minimally affected.

Serial sections of internal mammary arteries were analysed by Jülke et al. at Zürich University (1989) in a prospective series of 48 necropsy cases. Various degrees of luminal narrowing expressed as percentage of occluded surface area in relation to total surface area inside of the internal lamina elastica of the internal mammary artery were found; a normal internal mammary artery from this series is shown in Fig. 9. There is no intimal thickening in this specimen (mean thickness of endothelium and subendothelial collagen accounts for only 2.5 μm in comparison to a lumen diameter of more than 1000 μm; see also Sect. 3.1) and therefore luminal narrowing is almost 0%. A sample with luminal narrowing between 0% and 25% is shown in Fig. 23. The intimal thickening occludes 15% of the surface inside of the lamina elastica interna. The microscopic view of more severe luminal narrowing is shown in Fig. 24 where the occluded area accounts for 53%. Further analyses showed that atherosclerosis in the internal mammary arteries occured later and if, at a lesser degree, than in the coronary arteries of the same patient.

Sections of the distal end of the left internal mammary artery were analysed prospectively in a series of 32 patients undergoing coronary artery revascularization in collaboration with J. Cox, Geneva. These microscopic studies of the internal mammary artery showed:

- normal arterial wall in 22 patients (67%)
- minimal endofibrosis in 9 patients (27%)
- luminal narrowing less than 25% in 1 patient (3%)
- luminal narrowing between 25% and 50% in 1 patient (3%)
- luminal narrowing of more than 50% in no patient

A more detailed prospective study is still in progress to achieve higher patient numbers and more reliable results.

These data, together with the angiographic data, support the routine use of the internal mammary artery for coronary artery revascularization. However, anatomical variations and pathological lesions of the internal mammary arteries do occur and therefore careful evaluation of the internal mammary arteries has to be recommended in any patient in whom the use of these vessels is contemplated. Routine angiography of the subclavian arteries and the internal mammary arteries during coronary catheterization appears to be a useful tool for preoperative evaluation of these vessels.

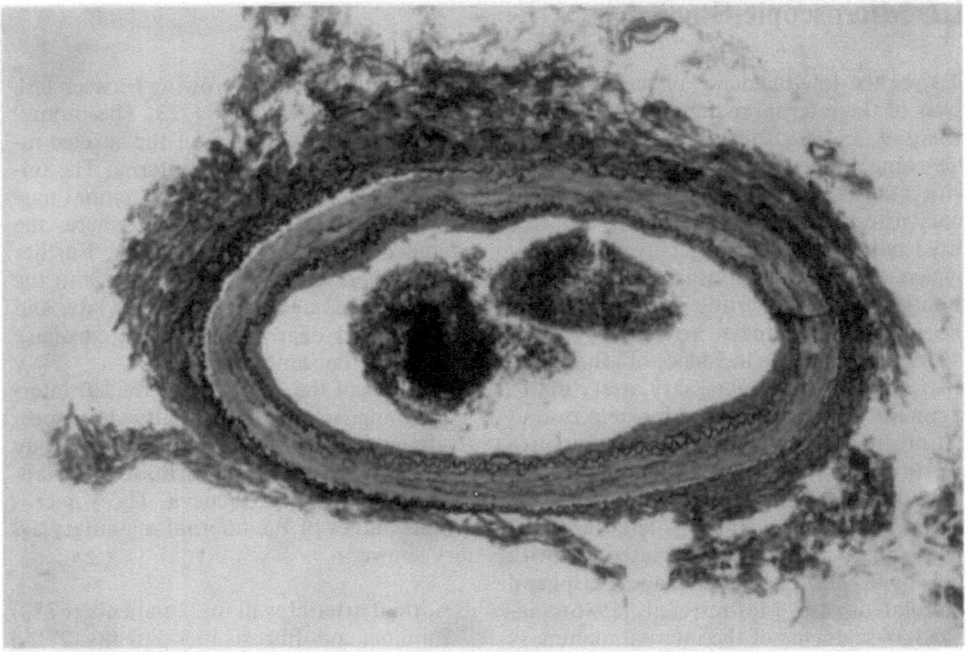

Fig. 23. Microscopic view of an internal mammary artery section with luminal narrowing of 15% due to intimal hyperplasia (van Gieson)

Fig. 24. Microscopic view of an internal mammary artery section with luminal narrowing of 53% due to severe intimal hyperplasia (van Gieson)

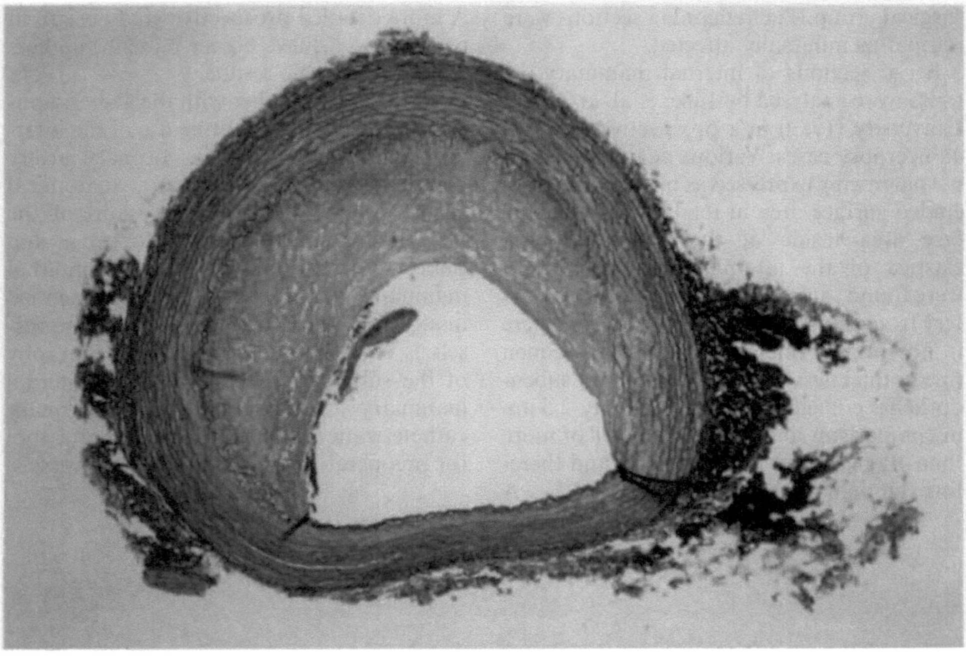

5 Experimental Studies

5.1 Flow Studies in Animals

5.1.1 Normal Internal Mammary Artery Flow

Internal mammary artery flow studies had already been performed at the time of Vineberg's operation when the internal mammary artery was implanted into the myocardium (Blesovsky et al. 1967; William-Olson et al. 1968; William-Olson 1971; Yokoyama et al. 1972; Bloomer et al 1973). In 1968 Wakabayashi and Connolly reported comparative flow studies of myocardial revascularization grafts. They analyzed two groups of dogs, one with indirect myocardial revascularization (implantation of the internal mammary artery in a myocardial tunnel) and one with direct myocardial revascularization (implantation of a vein or the internal mammary artery between the aorta and a coronary artery) and showed that mean flow through the direct coronary artery bypass grafts increased about twofold when the coronary artery was occluded.

McCormick et al. reported in 1975 on blood flow and vasoactive drug effects (isoproterenol, phenylephrine, and epinephrine) in internal mammary artery grafts and venous bypass grafts implanted onto the coronary arteries in mongrel dogs. Blood flow through vein grafts and internal mammary artery grafts was similar under basal conditions and increased similarly with each of the tested vasoactive agents.

Flow capacity of the canine internal mammary artery was reported in 1986 by Chuen-Neng et al. In situ blood flow in the internal mammary artery was 27 ml/min. Blood flow was 63 ml/min in the circumflex coronary artery and 42 ml/min in the left anterior descending coronary artery. After anastomosis of the left internal mammary artery to the circumflex coronary artery, the left main coronary artery was ligated; flow through the bypass graft increased to 92 ml/min and systemic hemodynamics remained stable. Isoproterenol stimulation further increased flow through the left internal mammary artery graft to 160 ml/min. The authors concluded that the canine internal mammary artery is capable of substantial early increase in flow and can, in fact, support the entire left coronary circulation.

5.1.2 Internal Mammary Artery Flow and Vasoactive Drugs

The internal mammary artery graft is a dynamic graft (Singh and Sosa 1984), wheras the saphenous vein graft is passive. Therefore, potential exists not only for beneficial vasodilatation but also for spasm of this artery, which may be catastrophic. Vasoactive drug effects on blood flow in internal mammary artery and saphenous vein grafts were analyzed by Jett et al. (1987) in a canine right heart bypass preparation. Both the internal mammary and saphenous vein grafts were constructed so that they perfused the same coronary artery bed. The results suggested that flow through the canine internal mammary artery is changed by the drugs commonly used in perioperative management. Epinephrine and nitroglycerin increased internal mammary artery flow and decreased saphenous vein graft flow whereas nitroprusside had the opposite effect. The authors concluded that the vascular reactivity of the internal mammary artery must be considered when these drugs are used after coronary revascularization.

The response of the canine internal mammary artery graft to vasoactive drugs was also analyzed by Beavis et al. (1988). After anastomosis to the left anterior descending coronary artery, the authors analyzed its response to epinephrine, metaraminol, isoproterenol and calcium. Blood flow in the internal mammary artery clearly paralleled changes in systolic blood pressure with perfusion pressure being of prime importance in maintaining flow in the internal mammary artery. No deleterious effect of systemic vasoconstricting agents was demonstrated under normovolemic conditions.

5.1.3 Internal Mammary Artery Flow Under Pathological Hemodynamic Conditions

Internal mammary artery grafts deliver initially less flow to the coronary arteries in comparison to saphenous vein grafts (Flemma et al. 1975) and this lower flow can be reduced even more due to spastic reactions of the internal mammary artery (von Segesser et al. 1987b). The present study (von Segesser et al. 1989[1]) has been designed to evaluate the internal mammary artery flow isolated from the coronary artery bed as a function of different hemodynamic situations as they can occur following coronary artery bypass surgery (e.g., with severe bleeding, arrhythmia, low output) and as a function of various pharmacological interventions.

5.1.3.1 Material and Methods

The study included ten mongrel dogs with a body weight of 19 ± 5 kg (mean ± standard deviation). General anesthesia was induced with pentothal and maintained with volatile anesthetics. After median sternal splitting incision the right internal mammary artery was taken down with a muscular pedicle by combined low power cautery and ligation. Then the pericardium was opened and the right atrium exposed. Continuous recording of ECG (heart rate), central venous pressure, pulmonary artery pressure (wedge pressure), and arterial pressure was performed with a seven-channel Gould recording system. Cardiac output was assessed by thermodilution (Edwards) at regular intervals. An electromagnetic flow probe (Biotronex) was placed at the origin of the internal mammary artery. After measurement of free internal mammary artery flow (volumetric tank and timer) and calibration of the flow meter (Biotronex) the distal end of the internal mammary artery was implanted onto the right atrial appendage end-to-side with a 7/0 monofilament polypropylene continuous suture and a 24 G Teflon catheter connected to a pressure measuring line and a Statham transducer was installed 4 cm above the distal end of the internal mammary artery.

This model, with the internal mammary artery dissected free as a pedicle and implanted onto the right atrium, allows one to study the effects of various conditions on the isolated internal mammary artery and independently from the coronary artery bed.

Hemodynamic Studies

The hemodynamic parameters mentioned above, including internal mammary artery flow and distal internal mammary artery pressure, were analyzed for the following situations:

- normovolemia and steady state
- sudden hypovolemia (withdrawal of 20% of calculated circulating blood volume over 90 s)
- gradual hypovolemia (withdrawal of 20% of calculated circulating blood volume over 240 s)
- bolus of nitrates (Perlinganit 500 μg/kg)
- bolus of epinephrine (5 μg/kg)
- severe hypovolemia and bolus of epinephrine (5 μg/kg)

Measurements were performed continuously wherever possible and read every 60 s during and after intervention, till stabilization of hemodynamics occurred. After administration of each agent, sufficient time was allowed for restitution of the preadministration hemodynamic values. Hypovolemia was corrected by retransfusion of the withdrawn volume.

Data Analyses

Quantitative data are presented as the mean ± standard deviation. Comparison of quantitative data is made using Student's t-test for paired variables where appropriate. Statistical significance is confirmed by the probability value $\mathbf{P} < 0.05$.

[1] Reprinted with permission from the Society of Thoracic Surgeons (*The Annals of Thoracic Surgery*, Vol 47: 575–579, 1989)

5.1.3.2 Results

Continuous registration (pulsatile mode) of internal mammary artery flow, arterial pressure, central venous pressure, ECG, pulmonary artery pressure, and distal internal mammary artery pressure is shown in Fig. 25. The synchronous pulses of arterial pressure, internal mammary artery pressure, and the consecutive pulsatile internal mammary artery flow are documented. Figure 26 shows the continuous registration of the

Fig. 25. Continuous registration (pulsatile mode) of hemodynamics under normovolemic conditions (ECG, central venous pressure, pulmonary artery pressure, and arterial pressure) and hemodynamics of the internal mammary artery (IMA; distal IMA pressure and IMA flow). Paper speed 25 mm/s

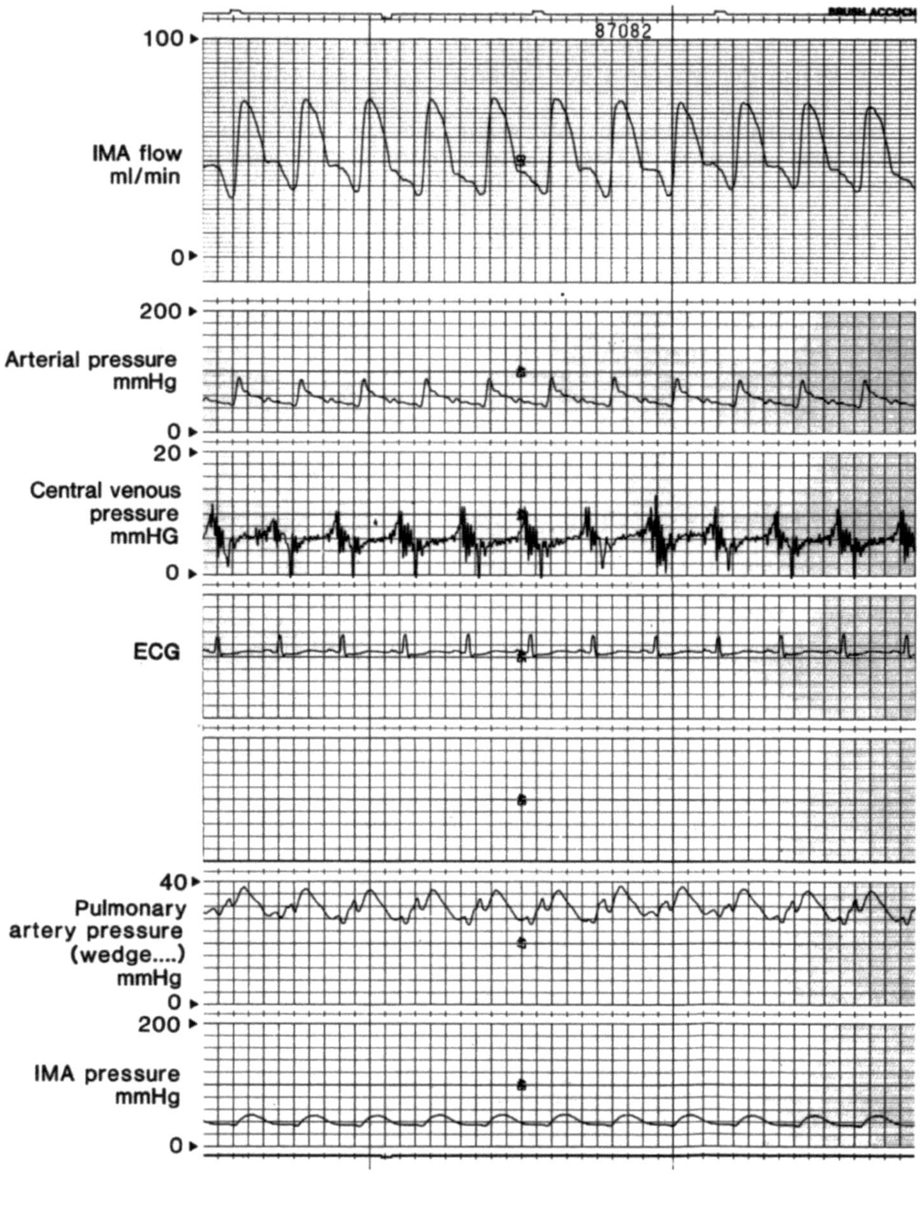

hemodynamics (mean mode) during fast withdrawal of 20% of the calculated circulating blood volume (sudden hypovolemia: period *A*, 90 s), stabilization (period *A*–*B*) and retransfusion (period *B*, 240 s) of the same blood volume. During hypovolemia the internal mammary artery flow drops to almost 0 whereas the arterial pressure, measured in the aorta, and the pressure in the internal mammary artery drop to about 50% (period *A*). There is a slight recovery of all curves during stabilization and progressive recovery during retransfusion (period *B*) of the withdrawn volume. After retransfusion all recorded parameters reach almost the baseline values.

Serial studies in ten animals with sudden hypovolemia are given in Table 1. For a mean reduction of cardiac output from 3.3±0.8 l/min to 2.2±0.9 (−33%) the aortic pressure drops from 94±22 mmHg to 48±4 (−49%) and distal internal mammary artery pressure drops from 71±20 mmHg to 33±9 (−54%) whereas internal mammary artery flow drops from 66±30 ml/min to 10±9 (−85%). The differences measured before and after withdrawal of the predetermined volume are highly significant for all parameters (Table 1).

The values of the other analyzed conditions are given in Table 2. Gradual hypovolemia (withdrawal of the same amount of blood as in sudden hypovolemia, but over a longer period, 240 s) shows less dramatic effects. During the observation period the aortic pressure dropped from 85±15 mmHg to 55±14 (−35%) and internal mammary artery flow dropped from 71±16 ml/min to 34±16 (−51%).

Similar effects are observed after administration of high doses of nitrates as bolus.

Table 1. Sudden Hypovolemia. Measurements performed 120 s after onset of withdrawal of volume or 30 s after completed withdrawal of volume (20% of calculated circulating blood volume over 90 s)

	Baseline	Shock	Change	P
Heart rate	138±20	154±20	+ 12%	< 0.01
Right atrial pressure (mmHg)	7±2	6±2	− 17%	< 0.01
Pulmonary artery pressure (mmHg)	15±6	12±5	− 20%	< 0.001
Wedge pressure (mmHg)	10±5	7±3	− 30%	< 0.001
Aortic pressure (mmHg)	94±22	48±4	− 49%	< 0.001
Cardiac output (l/min)	3.3±0.8	2.2±0.9	− 33%	< 0.001
Distal IMA pressure (mmHg)	71±20	33±9	− 54%	< 0.001
IMA flow (ml/min)	66±30	10±9	− 85%	< 0.001

Table 2. Other conditions. Gradual hypovolemia: Withdrawal of 20% calculated circulating blood volume over 240 s. Nitrates: Perlinganit 500 µg/kg bodyweight bolus. Epinephrine: 5 µg/kg bodyweight bolus. Severe hypovolemia + epinephrine: 5 µg/kg bodyweight bolus

	Interval (s)	Aortic pressure (mmHg)	IMA pressure (mmHg)	IMA flow (ml/min)
Normovolemia	0	85±15	67±17	71±16
Gradual hypovolemia	120	60±6	45±11	50±21
	240	55±14	39±14	34±16
Normovolemia	0	94±10	76±12	117±60
Nitrates	60	49±7	30±7	34±10
Normovolemia	0	70±5	58±8	88±13
Epinephrine	60	85±5	70±10	138±13
Severe hypovolemia	0	45±5	30±5	30±20
Epinephrine	60	48±7	34±4	18±12

For an aortic pressure drop from 94±10 mmHg to 49±7 (−48%) the internal mammary artery flow dropped from 117±60 ml/min to 34±10 (−71%).

Injection of epinephrine bolus under normovolemic conditions provoked a slight increase of aortic pressure from 70±5 mmHg to 85±5 (+21%) and also a marked in-

Fig. 26. Continuous registration (mean mode) of hemodynamics during sudden hypovolemia (period **A**, 90s), stabilization (period **A–B**), and retransfusion (period **B**). Mechanical zero of IMA flow probe is checked twice during period **A–B** and once at the end of period **B** (no modification). Wedge pressure is measured at the end of period **A**, at the end of period **A–B**, and during period **B**. Paper speed 1 mm/s

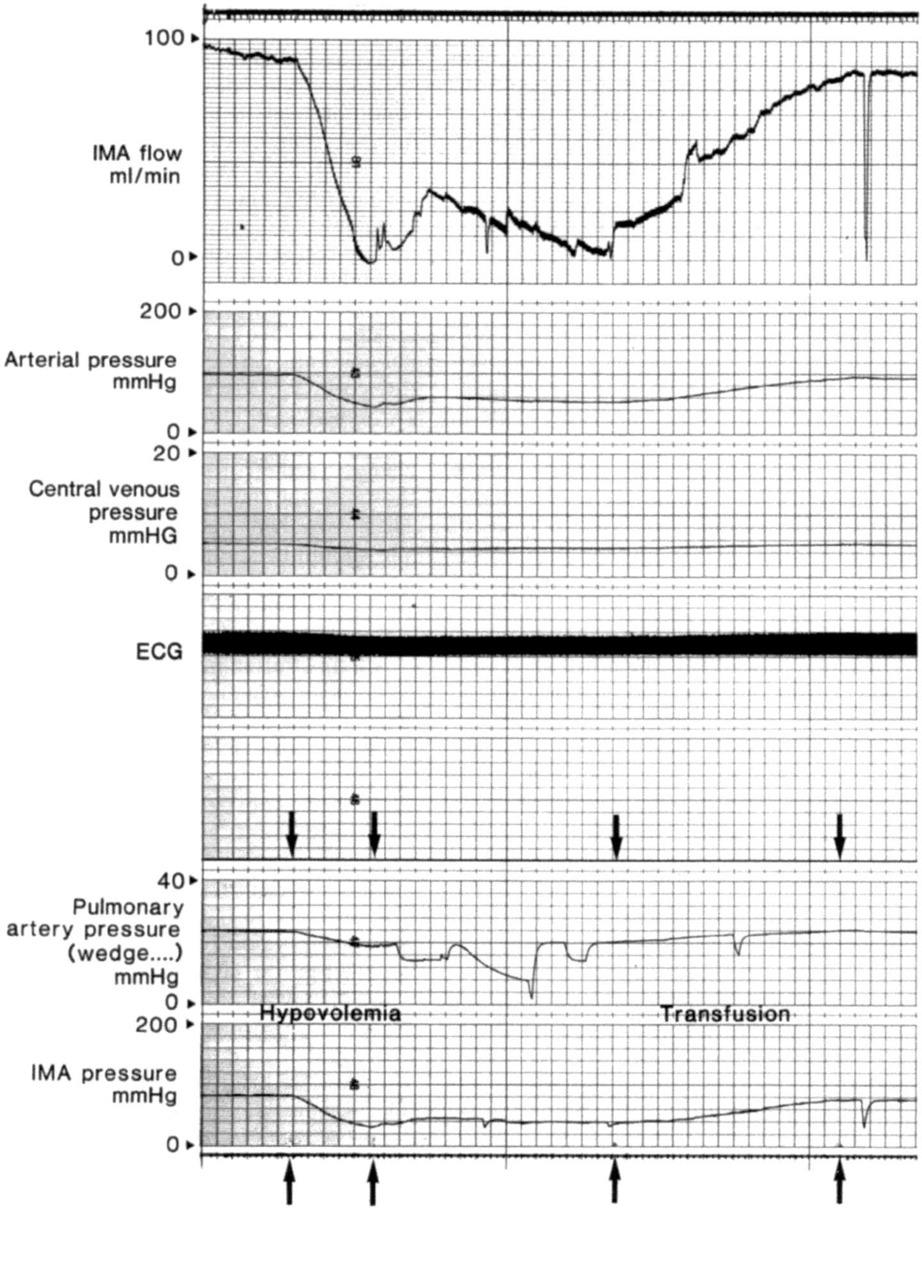

crease of internal mammary artery flow from 88±13 ml/min to 138±13 (+57%). Under sudden hypovolemia, however, administration of epinephrine bolus provoked only a minimal increase of the aortic pressure from 45±5 mmHg to 48±7 (+7%) and a contrasting decrease of internal mammary artery flow from 30±20 ml/min to 18±12 (−40%).

5.1.3.3 Discussion

Hypovolemic shock led to disproportionate internal mammary artery flow reduction in the canine model as documented in Fig. 26 and demonstrated for serial analyses ($n = 10$) in Table 1 where the internal mammary artery flow drop was 85% as a function of an aortic pressure drop of 49%. The pressure difference between the two ends of the internal mammary artery (aortic pressure − central venous pressure) was 87 mmHg before hypovolemia and 42 mmHg after hypovolemia (change pressure 52%). Therefore the internal mammary artery flow drop is also disproportionate in comparison to the pressure difference before and after hypovolemia. This reaction can be explained by the stress-induced α-adrenergic sympathetic stimulation, i.e., release of norepinephrine, and triggering of other vasoactive mediators, provoking peripheral vasoconstriction. It has been shown that the internal mammary artery is a living conduit (Singh and Sosa 1984) which will react with vasoconstriction after α-adrenergic stimulation.

Disproportionate flow reduction of the internal mammary artery used as the graft for coronary artery revascularization can have deleterious effects in critical situations, e.g., weaning from cardiopulmonary bypass (von Segesser et al. 1987 b), and especially in patients with few collaterals as may occur after resection of coronary artery aneurysms (von Segesser et al. 1987 c).

After retransfusion and stabilization, gradual hypovolemia provoked by withdrawal of the same amount of blood over a period of 240 s instead of 90 s shows less dramatic effects with an aortic pressure drop of 35% and a nearly proportionate reduction in internal mammary artery flow of 51%. The difference observed between sudden hypovolemia and gradual hypovolemia can be explained by the lack of time for adequate autoregulation in the former situation.

Massive bolus injection of nitrates led to a reaction similar to gradual hypovolemia: the aortic pressure drop of 59% is in the same range as the internal mammary artery flow drop of 71%. It can be speculated that the relatively proportionate drops are either due to the vasodilating effects of the nitrates, the relatively gentle secondary onset of hypovolemia, or both.

Epinephrine bolus under normovolemic conditions led to a significant increase of internal mammary artery flow (+57%, $P < 0.05$). This effect is due to the positive chronotropic and positive inotropic effects of high doses of epinephrine and the consecutive increase of cardiac output. Increased internal mammary artery flow under normovolemic conditions has been previously documented in other studies where the internal mammary arteries were implanted onto the coronary arteries (McCormick et al. 1975, Beavis et al. 1988). However, those studies did not separate the vasomotor changes in the coronary vascular bed from those in the internal mammary arteries. These two beds represent serial resistors, and should be studied independently to determine the relative contribution of each segment to the observed changes in internal mammary artery flow.

Administration of epinephrine bolus after severe hypovolemia provoked, as expected, some increase of aortic pressure (+7%). However, when hypovolemia is very severe and epinephrine doses are high enough, the slight increase of aortic pressure appears to be mainly due to extreme vasoconstriction as documented by a decrease of internal mammary artery flow (−40%). This situation might be difficult to overcome if coronary artery blood flow is predominantly supplied by the internal mammary arteries.

We are aware of the fact that these analyses were performed with extreme volume shifts and high doses of vasoactive drugs. However, in this study, we were dealing with a healthy myocardium in contrast to clinical practice where, when problems occur, the myocardial activity might be termed: "weak action", and little or no response can be expected after application of positive inotropic agents. We conclude, that sudden severe hypovolemia can lead to disproportionate internal mammary artery flow reduction and that pharmacological interventions are difficult under these circumstances.

5.2 Physiological and Pathophysiological Basis for the Superiority of Internal Mammary Artery Grafts in Comparison to Saphenous Vein Grafts

Many factors that might be responsible for the superiority of the internal mammary artery as a graft material for coronary artery revascularization in comparison to the saphenous vein have been proposed in the past. They include utilization of an arterial graft for an arterial revascularization instead of an arterialized venous graft, the use of an active, "live" conduit (Singh and Sosa 1984) with intact vasomotricity (von Segesser et al. 1989) instead of a passive venous conduit, the use of a conduit with superior wall elasticity in comparison to veins allowing the propagation of the pulse wave and reduction of intimal hyperplasia, the use of a graft with a pedicle instead of a naked vein without lymphatic drainage and vasa vasorum, and better size match with the internal mammary artery which, at the level of the anastomoses has about the same diameter as the coronary arteries in comparison to saphenous veins which have in general double the diameter or quadruple the surface area.

Dobrin et al. (1977) have analyzed the physiological basis for differences in flow with the internal mammary artery in comparison to the saphenous vein. The grafts (human) were analyzed in a tissue bath and pressurized. At 100 mmHg, internal mammary artery diameter was 2.7±0.2 mm ($n = 9$) and saphenous vein diameter was 4.7±0.2 mm ($n = 39$). Mean wall thickness was 0.26 mm for the internal mammary arteries and 0.39 mm for the saphenous veins.

Based on these data, at any volume flow, flow velocities in internal mammary arteries were computed to be three times those in saphenous veins. Reynolds numbers computed for internal mammary artery and saphenous vein diameter indicated that flow in bypass grafts is probably nonturbulent. At 100 mmHg, activation of the vascular muscle elicited a 15% decrease in diameter of the internal mammary arteries, but only a 3% decrease in diameter of the saphenous veins. In related studies, steel tubes 0.84–4.39 mm inner diameter were perfused with human blood to measure the pressure drop with flow. For flows up to 200 ml/min, pressure drop was minimal with decreasing diameter until 2–3 mm was reached. At this diameter pressure drop increased sharply. Integration of flow-pressure loss data for the internal mammary artery and the saphenous vein diameters showed that the cumulative pressure loss along the course of the internal mammary arteries results in decreased exit pressure to perfuse native coronary vessels. This provides a quantitative physiological explanation for the lower coronary flows obtained clinically with the internal mammary arteries as compared with the saphenous veins.

Superior handling during take down of the internal mammary artery, which remains perfused until the very last moment before implantation onto the coronary artery unlike the harvesting of the saphenous vein, which has to be flushed with blood, saline, or other solutions and is often stored for a significant time at room temperature appears to be another important factor as shown by Lehmann et al. (1988). Figure 27 shows the scanning electron micrograph of the distal end of an internal mammary artery which was taken down by routine, low power electrocautery, with an intact endothelial layer. Figure 28 shows the contrasting surface of a saphenous vein, harvested with standard techniques and flushed with blood. In the latter the endothelial surface viewed is in poor shape. Sampling was performed immediately before anastomosis for both grafts; the scanning electron micrographs were performed by the Divison of

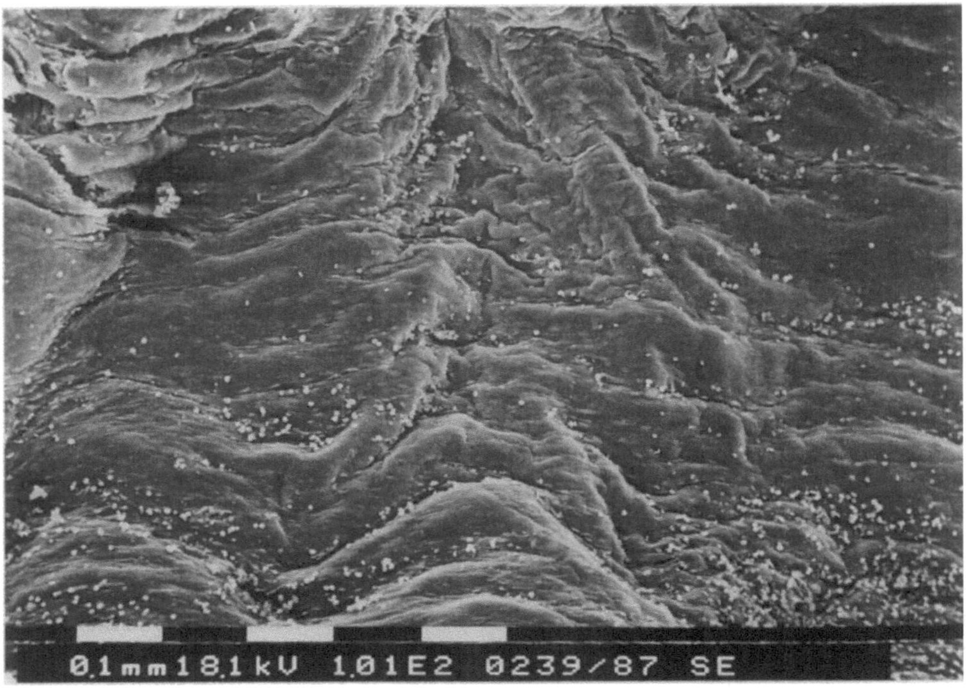

Fig. 27. Scanning electron microscopic view of the inner surface of an internal mammary artery after take-down: intact endothelium (**white bar** represents 100 μm)

Fig. 28. Scanning electron miroscopic view of the inner surface of a saphenous vein after harvesting by standard technique: damaged endothelial layer (**white bar** represents 100 μm)

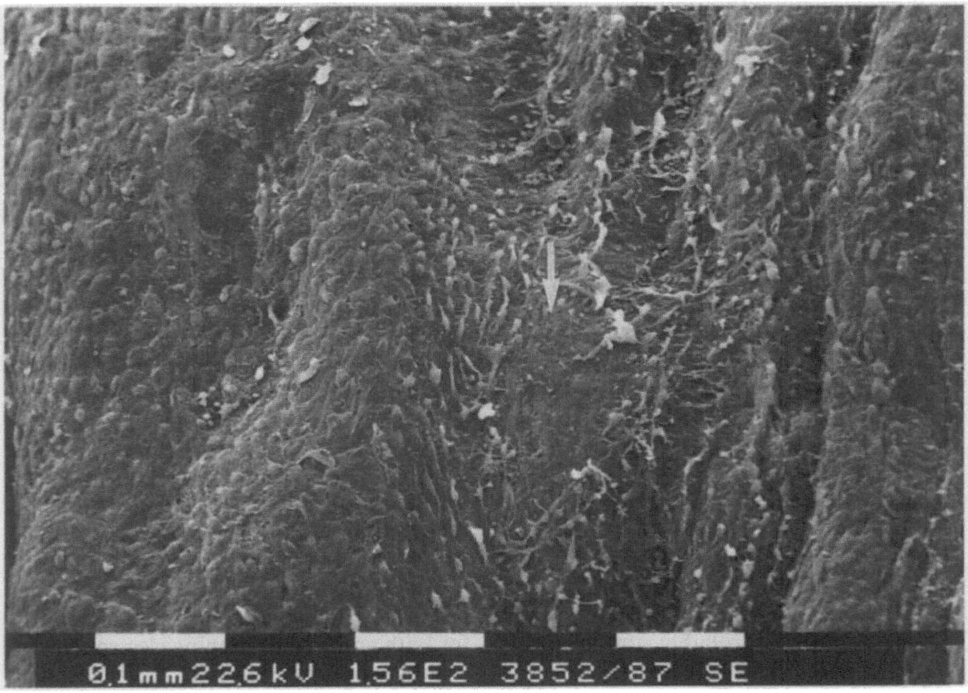

Cell Biology, Department of Anatomy Zürich University.

Loss of endothelium exposes the intima to the circulating blood elements and compounds. Early aggregation of platelets in vein grafts may release (through contact with collagen) a factor that promotes smooth muscle proliferation and migration (Ross et al. 1974), an integral part of the intimal hyperplasia–atherosclerosis complex. Platelets also release vasoactive substances, such as thromboxane A_2, which activate further aggregation, and the clotting mechanism, leading to a fibrin–platelet clot (Hamberg et al. 1974). Reduced fibrinolytic activity of transplanted veins (Malone et al. 1981) and impaired release of endothelium-derived relaxing factor (Angelini et al. 1989) have also been reported.

5.2.1 Internal Mammary Arteries and Prostacyclin Production

The importance of intact endothelium in the prevention of intravascular thrombosis was established by Virchow. One important factor in the remarkable antithrombotic function of the endothelium seems to be the production of prostacyclin (prostaglandin I_2) a potent vasodilator and inhibitor of platelet aggregation (Moncada and Vane 1980). Prostacyclin is the natural antagonist of thromboxane A_2, a platelet released vasoconstrictor and activator of platelet aggregation. Prostacyclin is labile and hydrolyzes spontaneously to the stable but inactive 6-keto-prostaglandin F_1. Prostacyclin production of internal mammary arteries and saphenous veins was studied by Chaikhouni et al. (1986) in 11 patients. Their observations suggested that the capacity of the internal mammary artery to produce prostacyclin in both a basal and a stimulated state is greater than that of the saphenous vein. These results are in accordance with the generally accepted finding that arteries produce more prostacyclin than veins (Skidgel and Printz 1978). However, the study does not permit one to separate the influence of potentially present endothelial damage due to the different preparation techniques for internal mammary arteries and saphenous veins (Lehmann et al 1988).

Prostacyclin production in free internal mammary artery grafts with and without surrounding tissue versus native internal mammary artery grafts with surrounding tissue was analyzed by Aarnio et al. (1988) in a series of eight dogs. Both types of free graft were anastomosed first to the left internal mammary artery one after another and then to the left anterior descending coronary artery. Harvesting was performed 6 months later and prostacyclin (prostaglandin I_2) production of the free internal mammary artery grafts and the intact internal mammary arteries was analyzed. This study showed that free internal mammary artery grafts were able to produce as much prostacyclin (prostaglandin I_2) as were control internal mammary artery grafts and that the type of dissection did not affect the result.

5.2.2 Endothelium-dependent Relaxations of the Internal Mammary Artery

Endothelium-dependent relaxations (Furchgott and Zawadzky 1980) in internal mammary arteries and saphenous veins obtained from patients undergoing coronary bypass surgery were analyzed by Lüscher et al. in Basel (1988). Rings with and without endothelium were suspended in organ chambers and isometric tension was recorded. Acetylcholine (10^{-8} to 10^{-4} M), thrombin (1 U/ml) and adenosine diphosphate (10^{-7} to 10^{-4} M) evoked potent endothelium-dependent relaxations in the internal mammary artery, but little or no responses in the saphenous vein ($\mathbf{P} < 0.005$). In the internal mammary artery, the relaxations were greatest with acetylcholine (98% ± 2%). The maximal response to thrombin was 44% ± 7% and to adenosin diphosphate 39% ± 8%. In the saphenous vein, the relaxations were below 15% with either agonist. Relaxation was unaffected by indomethacin (10^{-5} M), but was inhibited by methylene blue ($\mathbf{P} < 0.005$ and 0.01 respectively) and hemoglobin, indicating that the response was mediated by endothelium derived relaxing factor. Endothelium-independent relaxations to sodium nitroprusside were comparable in the mammary artery and the saphenous vein. The authors concluded that endothelium-dependent relaxations are greater in the internal mammary artery than in saphenous veins. Most probably nitric oxide (NO) accounts for the activity of the factor. Thus, endothelial cells produce endogenous nitrates causing vasodilation and inhibition of platelet adhesion and aggregation. These mechanisms may contribute to the higher patency rates of the internal mammary artery grafts in comparison to saphenous vein grafts.

5.2.3 Early Postoperative Changes of Saphenous Vein Grafts

Autologous vein grafts undergo many changes after operation both in the human and the experimental models (Brody et al. 1972; Fuchs et al. 1978). Most changes involve the intimal layer and include in the acute phase endothelial sloughing, edema, and deposition of fibrin, leukocytes, and platelets on the denuded surface.

In the early postoperative phase muscle necrosis and swelling of the media have also been noted in saphenous vein grafts. Regeneration of intima and media is by fibroblasts and smooth muscle cells. After a few weeks, endothelial cells cover the thickened intima (Fuchs et al. 1978). This fibrous replacement of the vein layers renders the graft rigid, noncompliant to the arterial pressure stress.

Fibrous thickening or intimal hyperplasia may be regarded as a sign of aging of the vessel wall, a phenomenon noted in the first year of life in human coronary arteries (Velican and Velican 1976). Arteries that do not show intimal thickening usually remain free of atheroma. Transplanted vein grafts lose their lymphatic drainage and vasa vasorum (McGeachy et al. 1981). Edema and thickening of the vein walls are a sign or a cause of poor transport of lymph and proteins filtering through the graft lumen (Grondin 1984). Enzymatic activity of the venous intima, which may differ from the arterial intima (DeMey et al. 1982; Aarnio 1988), and which regulates entry and clearance of lipids (Wolinsky 1980), fibrin (Malone et al. 1981), and other substances, is altered following transplantation in the arterial circuit as a result of trauma (Lehmann et al. 1988), hyperoxia, or the different hemodynamics (Grondin 1984). The sum of these and other modifications of saphenous vein grafts used for coronary artery revascularization results in the bypass attrition documented in Sect. 2.3.

5.3 Expanded Use of the Internal Mammary Artery

The superior results of revascularization of the left anterior descending coronary artery with the left internal mammary artery in comparison to the saphenous vein aortocoronary graft have led to a rapid increase in clinical use of the internal mammary artery, including isolated anastomoses to all main coronary arteries and their branches, sequential internal mammary artery anastomoses (Kabbani et al 1983; Harjola et al. 1984; Tector et al. 1984; Kamath et al 1985), internal mammary artery Y-graft (two terminal branches of the internal mammary artery are anastomosed (Tector et al. 1986)), anastomoses with the right internal mammary artery (Barner 1974a), anastomoses with both, right and left, internal mammary arteries (Lytle et al. 1986; Cosgrove et al. 1988) and all sorts of combinations. As there are only two internal mammary arteries available and as they are also limited in length it is difficult to reach the posterior wall and the distal coronary artery branches with this graft on one hand and on the other it is only rarely possible to perform complete revascularizations with the internal mammary arteries if three-vessel disease is present. Therefore, combinations of internal mammary artery grafts with saphenous vein grafts are necessary in most complex revascularization procedures. The experimental basis for this expansion based on extrapolating the results of the left internal mammary artery implanted onto the left anterior descending coronary artery, however, is poor.

Only a few alternatives have been evaluated in animal studies. One analyzed approach to expand the versatility of the internal mammary artery is the free aortocoronary internal mammary artery (clinically analyzed by Loop et al. 1986 b) that allows one to reach either distal coronary arteries, or several coronary artery branches to perform more sequential internal mammary artery coronary anastomoses. Another way to gain additional length is the use of the distally pedicled internal mammary artery with retrograde perfusion as suggested at the time of Vineberg's operation by Blesowsky et al. (1967) and Urschel and Morales (1967).

5.3.1 Free Internal Mammary Artery Grafts (Canine Experiments)

Free internal mammary artery grafts as canine femoral artery substitutes have been analyzed by Aarnio (1988). Both left and right internal mammary arteries were dissected free in six dogs, the left together with 2 cm wide surrounding tissue and the right as a naked artery. Free internal mammary artery grafts (3 cm long) were anastomosed end-to-end to the femoral arteries as femorofemoral graft. At 6 months all grafts were patent. Intimal thickening was seen in one graft on each side. Medial fibrosis was more common in the internal mammary artery grafts with surrounding tissue. Scanning electron microscopy showed endothelium in all grafts, but with some degeneration of endothelial cells. Instead of the normal spindle shape they were round. The cells showed dissociation and some sloughing. The author concluded that in free internal mammary artery grafts maintenance of patency was good. After retention in the femoral position for 6 months, the internal mammary artery grafts showed some morphological changes, which did not influence patency. Removal of surrounding tissue together with the internal mammary artery did not affect the outcome. The same author (Aarnio et al. 1988) has also analyzed the prostacyclin production in free internal mammary artery grafts with and without surrounding tissue in comparison to the native internal mammary artery in eight dogs (see Sect. 5.2.1). There was no significant difference between the free internal mammary artery grafts with and without surrounding tissue in comparison to the native internal mammary artery.

Patency and histologic structure of in situ internal mammary artery grafts, free internal mammary artery grafts, stripped, free internal mammary artery grafts, and stripped, free superficial femoral artery grafts were analyzed by Daly et al. (1988) in a canine model of coronary artery bypass ($n = 24$). Three months postoperatively, graft patency was assessed by angiogram and postmortem specimens were studied by intraluminal injection of a dilute barium solution proximal to the graft as well as microscopically. In situ internal mammary artery grafts and free internal mammary artery gafts were not significantly different in regard to patency, vascular wall cellular structure, or perfusion of the vasa vasorum. The stripped free internal mammary artery group had a higher incidence of thrombosis, intimal thickening, and medial injury than the pedicled (in situ and free internal mammary artery) grafts. The authors concluded that this difference may be due to early vascular wall ischemia as a result of poor early perfusion of the vasa vasorum. The stripped, free superficial femoral artery grafts were all patent, but had adventitial injury.

The three studies support the clinical use of the pedicled free internal mammary artery graft whereas the influence of surrounding tissue in internal mammary artery grafts remains controversial. Furthermore, the presence of morphological changes of the intima after 6 months of implantation in the femoral position might indicate that the free internal mammary artery graft is eventually not as good as the in situ internal mammary artery graft (see also Sect. 5.4.1). Thrombosed veins as well as sectioned lymphatics and nerves in the free pedicle could be responsible for this.

5.3.2 Retrograde Internal Mammary Artery–Coronary Artery Anastomoses (Canine Experiments)

As reported previously, the distal thirds of the left anterior descending, left circumflex and right coronary artery systems are difficult to reach with proximally pedicled internal mammary artery grafts. In an effort to expand the utilization of the internal mammary artery even further, revascularization of the distal coronary artery branches by means of distally pedicled retrograde internal mammary arteries was experimentally evaluated (von Segesser et al. 1989c[2]). This study was undertaken because the retro-internal mammary artery is well supplied with blood by its attachments to the intercostal, epigastric and musculophrenic arteries (see Fig. 8).

5.3.2.1 Material and Methods

Retrointernal mammary artery–coronary artery anastomoses were performed in ten mongrel dogs with a mean weight of 38 ± 13 kg. After induction of general anesthesia the chest was entered through a median sternal splitting incison. ECG (Hewlett Packard), right atrial pressure, left atrial pressure and femoral artery pressure (Millar microtip pressure transducers) were monitored continuously and recorded with an eight-channel memory oscilloscope (Lucius & Baer MS 8010) and an eight-channel paper recorder (W&W 408). Both left and right internal mammary arteries were taken down by combined, low power, cautery and ligation of side branches, and diluted papaverine was applied on a wet sponge. Heparin (300 I.U./kg body weight) was given and after cavoaortic cannulation the pump oxygenator was connected. Pump flow was kept at 100 ml/min/kg body weight. One internal mammary artery was transected at the level of the fifth intercostal space (anterointernal mammary artery) and the other internal mammary artery was transected at it's origin at the level of the subclavian artery (retrointernal mammary artery). Flow measurements (free into a beaker and by means of electromagnetic Biotronex flowprobes) as well as pressure measurements were performed for both, anterointernal mammary arteries and retrointernal mammary arteries. Retrointernal mammary artery–coronary artery anastomoses onto the distal left anterior descending coronary artery, distal obtuse marginal branch of the left circumflex coronary artery and posterior descending branch of the right coronary artery (Fig. 29) were performed under moderate hypothermia and induction of complete standstill of the heart with cardioplegic solution (St. Thomas'). After reperfusion and rewarming the animals were weaned from cardiopulmonary bypass and stabilized. The retrointernal mammary artery was cross-clamped and the revascularized coronary artery was snared proximally to the anastomosis with the retrointernal mammary artery (Fig. 30, point 1). After documentation of significant ischemia (Fig. 30, between points 1 and 2) the cross-clamp of the retrointernal mammary artery was released (Fig. 30, point 2) and the modifications of the ECG and the pressures were documented again. Finally, the snare on the coronary artery was released to see if there was any further modification of the parameters mentioned above in relation to eventually insufficient coronary artery perfusion by means of the retrointernal mammary–coronary artery anastomoses.

[2] Reprinted with permission from the *Thoracic and Cardiovascular Surgeon*, Vol 37: 143–146, 1989

Fig. 29. Range of anterograde internal mammary arteries and retrograde internal mammary arteries for clinical coronary artery revascularization

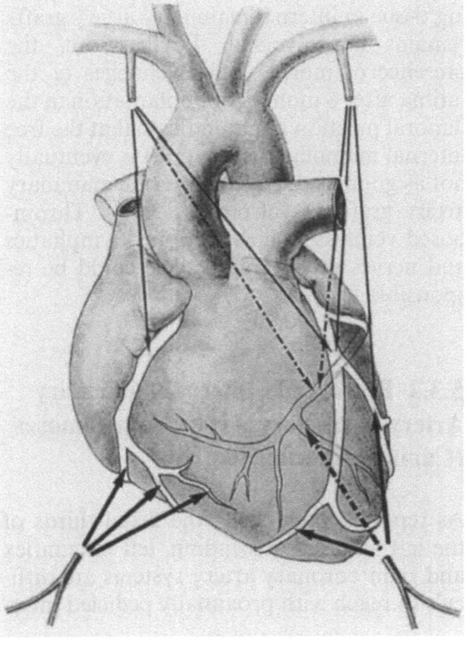

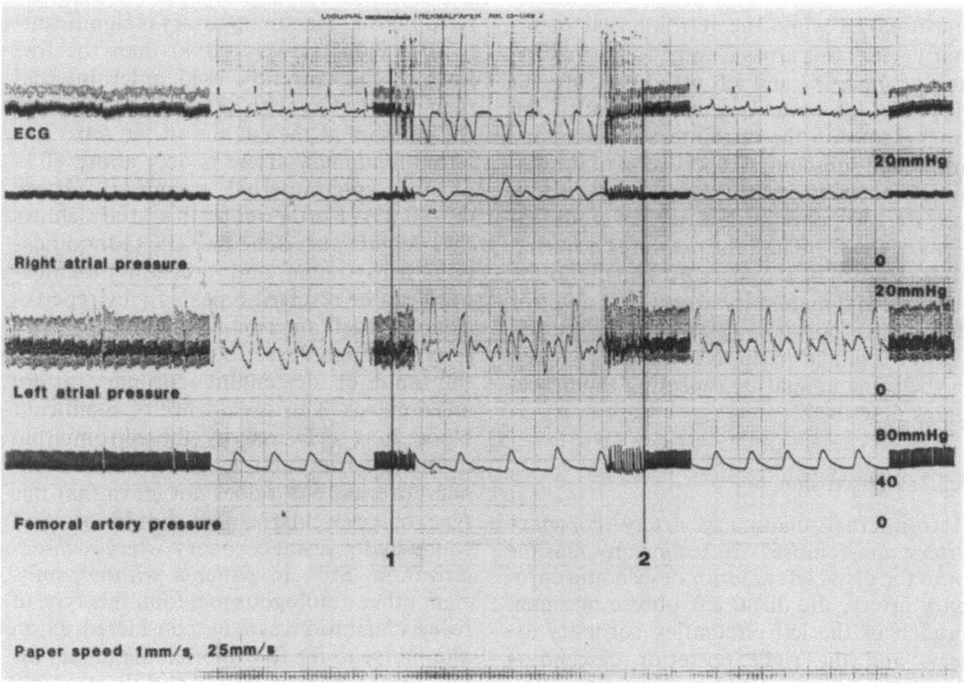

Fig. 30. Reversal of ischemia with retrointernal mammary artery. **Point 1**: Ligation of coronary artery proximal to retrointernal mammary artery–coronary artery anastomosis (retrointernal mammary artery cross-clamped): Ischemia. **Point 2**: Release of cross-clamp on the retrointernal mammary artery and reperfusion of the ligated coronary artery: Subsequent normalization of the monitored parameters

5.3.2.2 Results

At a mean systemic pressure of 68 ± 15 mmHg the mean pressure measured at the cut end of the internal mammary arteries with anterograde flow was 63 ± 14 mmHg in comparison to 50 ± 14 mmHg in the retrointernal mammary arteries with retrograde flow (**P** < 0.05; pressure ratio 0.8). With the same mean systemic pressure, mean anterograde free flow of the internal mammary arteries was assessed at 97 ± 43 ml/min in comparison to 48 ± 13 ml/min in the retrointernal mammary arteries with retrograde flow (**P** < 0.005; flow ratio 0.5).

The following retrointernal mammary artery–coronary artery anastomoses were performed (n = 10). Left retrointernal mammary artery–coronary artery anastomosis was established in six animals to the distal left anterior descending coronary artery and in two animals to the distal left obtuse marginal branch of the left circumflex coronary artery. Right retrointernal mammary artery–coronary artery anastomosis to the right posterior descending coronary artery was performed in two animals (see Fig. 29).

All animals could be weaned from cardiopulmonary bypass (10/10).

Functional blood supply of the left retrointernal mammary artery to the distal left anterior descending coronary artery was analyzed in the six animals with left retrointernal mammary artery–left anterior descending coronary artery anastomoses.

Significant ischemia with modification of the ECG and left atrial pressure, as documented in Fig. 30 point 1, could be provoked in 6/6 animals by ligation of the left anterior dscending coronary artery proximally to the retrointernal mammary artery–left anterior descending coronary artery anastomoses while the retrointernal mammary artery was cross-clamped. Normalization of the ECG and left atrial pressure occurred in 6/6 animals after removal of the cross-clamp on the retrointernal mammary artery and subsequent reperfusion of the distal left anterior descending coronary artery (see Fig. 30 point 2). No further modifications of the ECG and the pressures occurred after removal of the snare proximally to the retrointernal mammary artery–left anterior descending coronary artery anastomoses. However similar patterns could be provoked in the same animal by repeating the procedures described.

5.3.2.3 Discussion

Retrointernal mammary artery–coronary artery anastomoses are technically feasible onto the distal left anterior descending coronary artery, the distal left obtuse marginal branch of the left circumflex coronary artery, and the right posterior descending coronary arteries. Furthermore, retrointernal mammary artery–coronary artery anastomoses provide significant flow to the locally ischemic heart. Retrograde internal mammary artery implantation into the myocardium (Vineberg 1946) was reported in 1966, but despite the technical feasibility the pressure delivered by the retrointernal mammary artery was insufficient for durable patency in some and controversial in others (Blesovsky et al. 1967, Urschel and Morales 1967). Revascularization of the right coronary artery by retrograde perfusion of the mammary artery was analyzed in dogs by Florian et al. in 1975 with encouraging results. In 1980 Folts et al. reported successful use of the retrointernal mammary artery for revascularization of the canine circumflex artery. However, to the best of our knowledge, there is no comparative study on anterointernal mammary artery flow and retrointernal mammary artery flow in the literature, just as there is no report on retrointernal mammary artery–left anterior descending coronary artery anastomoses.

The present study shows that virtually all distal branches of the coronary arteries can be reached in the canine model with the distally pedicled retrointernal mammary artery. However, free backflow from the retrointernal mammary artery is significantly (**P** < 0.005) lower (50%) than the free flow of the currently used anterointernal mammary artery with anterograde flow and the pressure at the cut end of the retro-internal mammary artere is only about 80% of the anterointernal mammary artery (**P** < 0.05). Furthermore this study shows that significant ischemia (ECG-modification, arrhythmia, and pressure modification) can be reversed repeatedly by reperfusion of the left anterior descending coronary artery through the retrointernal mammary–left anterior descending coronary artery anastomosis. This is evidence of significant blood flow delivered by the retrointernal mammary artery to the ligated canine coronary arteries, but it does not mean that this type of revascularization should be used routinely for distal coronary artery revascularization. Still, in patients without sufficient other autologous material, this type of revascularization can be considered as an alternative to the free internal mammary artery graft (see Sect. 5.3.1) and the revascularization procedures by the splenic and epiploic arteries (see Sect. 5.4). This situation has previously occurred and retrointernal mammary artery–right posterior descending coronary artery anastomoses were performed during revascularization procedures in humans as reported in 1982 by Goiti and Smith, in 1986 by Livi et al., and in 1989 by Huttunen et al. There can be no doubt about substantial backflow through the distal collaterals of the internal mammary arteries in humans as probably all surgeons performing internal mammary-coronary artery anastomoses have some experience with persistent bleeding originating from these collaterals. However, the free flow of the human retrointernal mammary artery measured by Goiti et al. (1982) was only 40 ml/min and Livi et al. (1986) reported 60 ml/min. These figures account for a mean retrointernal mammary artery flow of 50 ml/min or only 36% of the 138 ml/min reported by Green (1971) as mean free flow for anterointernal mammary arteries in humans. Cohen et al. (1988) measured only 25 ± 17 ml/min for human retrointernal mammary arteries in comparison to 73 ± 34 ml/min for anterointernal mammary arteries. These results for the retrointernal mammary artery (retrograde flow 34% of anterograde flow) may be lower in comparison to other reports because the internal mammary arteries were transected only 5 mm above their bifurcation and were therefore supplied by only two collateral branches (see Fig. 8). The main indication for retrointernal mammary artery–coronary artery anastomoses might be patients with severely diseased ascending aorta and supraaortic vessels in combination with relatively distal coronary artery lesions.

In consideration of the reduced flow of the retrointernal mammary arteries in comparison to the anterointernal mammary arteries, as many collaterals as possible have to be preserved during the harvesting procedure in order to supply adequate flow (von Segesser et al. 1987b) to the revascularized coronary arteries.

5.4 Alternative Grafts for Coronary Artery Revascularization

To establish a valid alternative graft material for coronary artery revascularization was a major problem when the saphenous vein was the only graft used for coronary artery revascularization by 95% of surgeons. At that time it was difficult to find adequate autologous bypass material in patients with early ramification of the greater saphenous veins, in patients with major varicosities with or without vein stripping, in patients with phlebitis, and in patients in whom the saphenous veins had been removed for previous arterial reconstructions, especially in redo coronary artery revascularization. The lesser saphenous vein (Crosby and Craver 1975) can be successfully used for coronary artery revascularization. However, it can also show major varicosities or be unavailable for other reasons. Various biological and synthetic substitutes have been analyzed and have prooved to be inferior to the saphenous vein (Ulliot 1980) with one exception: the internal mammary artery.

5.4.1 Autologous Alternative Graft Materials

Besides the greater saphenous veins which have been used in thousands of patients for successful coronary artery revascularizations (Collins et al. 1973; Cameron et al. 1979; Loop et al. 1979; Kennedy et al. 1980; Braunwald 1983; Hahn 1983) and the lesser saphenous veins which have been used as complementarily, armveins have been used in the absence of sufficient saphenous veins. However, armveins have a much thinner vessel wall than saphenous veins and are known for accelerated attrition in the arterial environment (Schulman and Bradhey 1982). This might be due to the difference in hydrostatic pressure between the upper and the lower extremities due to the upright position of humans. The higher hydrostatic pressure in the saphenous veins, especially below the knee, might precondition the saphenous vein wall for the challenge of arterial perfusion.

Arterial autografts have been successfully used for arterial reconstruction, particularly in the aortorenal position, with normal growth of the graft (Stoney and Wilie 1970; Lye et al. 1975). But free radial grafts failed in coronary artery surgery (Carpentier et al. 1973; Curtis et al. 1975; Chiu 1976; Fisk et al. 1976, Loop et al. 1976). Gastroepiploic artery myocardial implants (Hirose et al. 1969) and splenic artery myocardial implants (Bloomer et al. 1973) have also been evaluated and were abandoned with Vineberg's operation.

No long term results in larger series are available for the recently reported use of the inferior epicastric artery as a free graft for myocardial revascularization (Puig et al. 1990) nor for the pedicled retro-internal mammary artery coronary artery bypass (von Segesser et al. 1989c).

In 1979, one case with coronary artery revascularization by a pedicled splenic artery was reported (Green et al. 1979). In 1987 two reports appeared on gastroepiploic–coronary artery anastomoses (Attum 1987, Pym et al. 1987). This type of revascularization has also been used at Zürich University with good early results. We have mainly used the route behind the stomach through the omental bursa to bring the pedicled right gastroepiploic artery to the diaphragm which is crossed through a median antero-posterior incision. The latter can later be enlarged at the proper level for optimal positioning of the pedicled graft. After weaning, the anterior part of the incision is readapted with some stitches as we are used to do in patients receiving extra-anatomic grafts from the ascending to the descending aorta.

In the meanwhile, several reports about the use of celiac trunk branches as coronary bypass grafts have been published. (Aarnio et al. 1989; Mills et al. 1989a; Suma et al. 1989 and Verkkala et al. 1989).

The experience reported by Mills and Everson (1989a) includes 39 patients undergoing coronary artery bypass grafting with the right gastroepiploic artery. Indications initially included poor quality or absent saphenous vein, ascening aortic atherosclerosis, and repeat coronary artery bypass grafting. Arteries bypassed with the right gastroepiploic artery were the posterior descending (22 patients), right coronary (12), diagonal (5), and marginal (4). Distal right gastroepiploic artery internal diameters of all grafts measured 1.5 to 3.25 mm (average diameter 2.14 mm). Pedicled graft lengths measured 18 to 30 cm (average length 23.7 cm), and free graft 8 to 24 cm (average length 17.7 cm). Early postoperative cardiac catheterization in 29 patients (19 pedicled and 10 free grafts) revealed all grafts to be patent without a kink or a twist, but three of the free right gastroepiploic artery grafts had vasospasm. Several routes have been used to bring the pedicled right gastroepiploic artery through the diaphragm as reported by Mills and Everson (1989b). Furthermore, multiple free (aorto-coronary) gastroepiploic coronary artery grafting has been reported since by Tanimoto et al. (1990). However, the place of the celiac trunk branches in clinical coronary artery revascularization has yet to be established. We have observed severe spastic reactions of the right gastroepiploic artery as well as significant stenoses of the celiac trunk and it's branches. The latter can occur even in younger patients with less than 45 years of age (von Segesser et al. 1986c). Hence we recommend angiographic visualization of the gastroepiploic artery prior to it's use for elective coronary artery revascularization. Further major concerns include abdominal complications, potential graft damage during future abdominal operations and the lacking long-term results.

5.4.2 Homologous Alternative Graft Materials

Homologous saphenous veins, either tanned or sterilized with antibiotic solutions, have been utilized in peripheral vascular surgery with moderate success. Application of these graft materials in coronary artery revascularization has been performed sporadically. A more recent approach is the use of cryopreserved saphenous vein grafts for coronary artery revascularization (Tice et al. 1976; Gelbfish 1986) in the absence of another more suitable autologous graft material. However, in the series reported by Gelbfish et al., 50% of the cryopreserved homologous saphenous veins ($n = 31$) were occluded at 1 year of follow-up. The authors concluded that use of cryopreserved homologous saphenous veins for coronary artery revascularization should be avoided if at all possible. No long-term results on reliable series are available up to now.

5.4.3 Biological Substitutes

Several biological grafts have been evaluated in clinical peripheral vascular surgery. Glutaraldehyde-preserved bovine arteries have been abandoned because of excessive aneurysm formation with increasing age. Somewhat better results have been obtained with tanned umbilical veins reinforced with a polyester mesh, but aneurysm formation is still present (Dardik et al. 1984, Hasson et al. 1986). Tanned collagenous tubes with ingrown polyester mesh, grown on mandrels implanted in sheep (Omniflo) and tanned bovine internal mammary arteries (Bioflow) are still under clinical evaluation.

None of the commercially available biological grafts equaled the saphenous vein graft in peripheral vascular reconstructive surgery (Largiadèr 1985) and only anecdotal reports on coronary artery revascularizations with these substitutes have been recorded.

Improved fixation techniques have been developed for better biological grafts which are made either from bovine internal mammary arteries or from bovine ureters (Flonova). But these grafts have to be evaluated in a number of trials before clinical application can be envisaged.

5.4.4 Synthetic Grafts

Synthetic grafts made from Dacron or Teflon have been widely used for peripheral arterial reconstruction. They provide acceptable results in the larger diameters. However, in revascularization of small vessels beyond the knee, they are much worse than saphenous vein grafts (von Segesser and Faidutti 1984, Largiadèr 1985). This has not been improved dramatically by the use of external supports and therefore other ways such as construction of sequential anastomoses and/or arterio-venous fistulas at the site of the distal anastomosis, to increase the graft flow, have been suggested.

In coronary artery revascularization expanded Teflon grafts have been used in exceptional situations. However no long term results of more than a few cases are available. Dacron tube grafts have been used systematically by Cabrol et al. (1986) for revascularization of the coronary arteries after implantation of a composite graft into the aortic root instead of direct reimplantation of the coronary artery ostia as reported by Bentall and de Bono (1968). Of course long term results of these complex procedures cannot be compared to those of isolated coronary artery revascularizations.

New materials such as polyurethanes, biodegradable or not, and plasma polymerized Teflon are still under investigation for peripheral vascular revascularization.

5.4.5 Grafts of the Future

Several grafts for coronary artery revascularization, or in more general terms for small vessel substitution are actually under development. The most promising appear to be the approaches looking for improved, more biocompatible surfaces exposed to the blood. This includes endothelial cell seeding

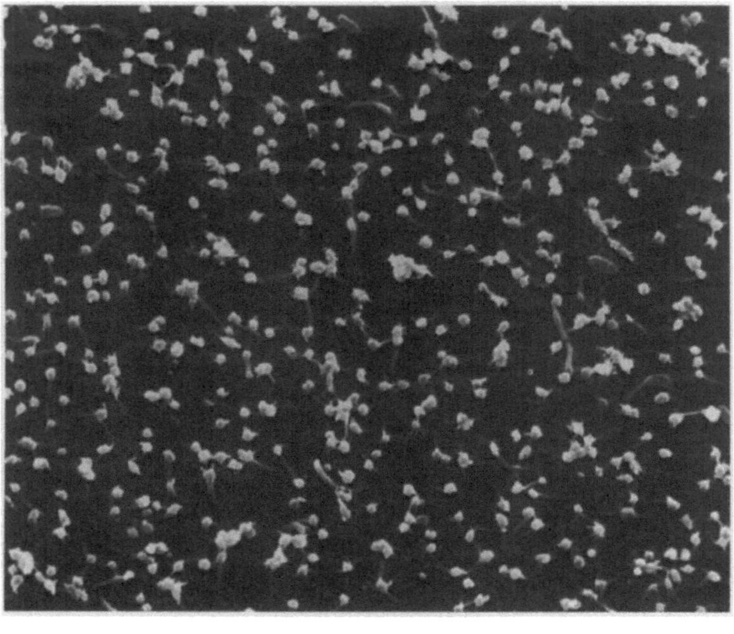

Fig. 31. Scanning electron micrograph of a heparin surface-coated tube after 6 hours of left heart bypass without systemic heparinization; no clots and only low grade activation of thrombocytes, as observed with full systemic heparinization. ×700

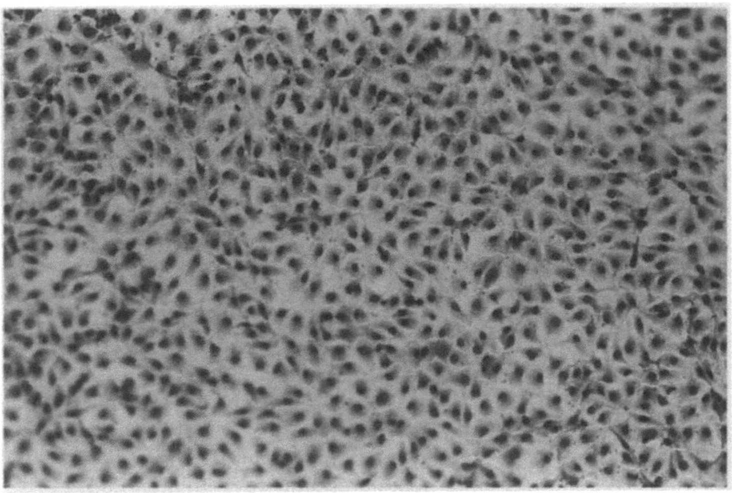

Fig. 32. Micrograph of a hybrid polyurethane graft with complete endothelial cell lining

or lining, heparin-like biomaterials and heparin surface coating.

The idea of heparin surface coating is not new. It was introduced by V. Gott in 1963 for the apicoaortic shunt which was applied clinically for the resection of aortic aneurysms without the need for systemic heparinization. In the meanwhile heparin surface coatings have been improved so far that open-chest cardiopulmonary bypass without systemic heparinization can be successfully realized in animal experiments (von Segesser and Turina 1989). Figure 31 shows a polyvinylchloride tube with heparin surface coating which was exposed to the blood during a 6-h left heart bypass without systemic heparinization. Only a few nonactivated thrombocytes and no clots are visible. Clinical application of heparin coated-membrane oxygenators for extracorporeal CO_2 removal has also been reported (Bindslev et al. 1987). Recently the concept of heparin surface coating has also been applied to biological grafts for coronary artery revascularization with interesting results in animal experiments (Nojiri et al. 1987).

A different and more complex approach is the realization of new grafts with endothelial cell lining of the entire bloodexposed surface. Müller et al. (1988) have realized a hybrid graft with near arterial compliance consisting of a polyurethane matrix with an inner, autologous, endothelial cell lining and an outer polyester mesh support. Figure 32 shows the inner surface of a hybrid graft with over 95% coverage by endothelial cells. These grafts show prostacyclin production similar to a vessel with its own endothelium. Initial animal experiments with femorofemoral implants are very promising.

6 Clinical Studies

6.1 Flow Studies in Humans

Several reports on internal mammary artery flow measured in humans have been published during the 20-year history of direct coronary artery revascularization. The flows measured in animals cannot be directly applied to humans as pointed out by Barner in 1987. In the studies of Lee et al. (1986) where the canine left internal mammary artery supplied the entire left-sided myocardial circulation when the left main coronary artery was ligated, the internal diameter of the internal mammary artery at the site of the anastomosis was 2.6 mm versus an average internal mammary artery diameter at the anastomosis of 2.0 mm or less in humans. Normal myocardial mass in a 70 kg man is about 350 g versus 250 g in the average 30 kg dog, and total coronary artery flow is somewhat greater in humans. Thus, in the experimental situation, the conduit is relatively much larger with correspondingly higher flow capacity and the myocardial mass is significantly less.

A number of human coronary graft flow data are shown in Table 3. The highest internal mammary artery flow measured with high accuracy is free internal mammary artery flow. Green et al. (1967) reported for the cut end of the human internal mammary artery a mean flow of 60–260 ml/min and a mean flow of 138 ml/min. One has to remember here that the internal mammary artery is a "life" conduit with its own reactions to dissection, cross-clamping, vasoactive drugs, hemodynamics in general, and maybe even nonpulsatile perfusion with the pump oxygenator. Therefore, an internal mammary artery has not one typical flow rate, but everything between zero and a maximum value.

Evaluation of flow rates after anastomosis of the internal mammary artery to the coronary arteries is even more complex. Not only the flow-determining parameters of the internal mammary artery have now to be taken in account, but also those of the recipient coronary vascular bed. This, and the still far from perfect measuring equipment, might explain the appreciable scatter of the measured internal mammary artery flows. The internal mammary artery graft flow after anastomosis to the coronary artery vessels measured with electomagnetic flow meters and calculated as a mean of the reported data is around 54 ml/min wheras the flow in saphenous vein aortocoronary grafts is about 79 ml/min (Table 3). These values were obtained with open-chest after weaning for cardiopulmonary bypass. A very interesting study on comparative hemodynamic properties of vein and mammary artery in coronary bypass operations was performed by Flemma et al. in 1975. To understand better the observed differences in bypass flows between the two grafts, a technique was devised for anastomosing both vein and internal mammary artery to the same anterior descending coronary artery (V-graft) in 14 patients. In the stable postperfusion state, flows in the two bypass conduits were simultaneously recorded as well as pressure relationships in both grafts and the left ventricle. The supply/demand ratio for left ventricular performance was calculated with respect to the diastolic pressure-time index/tension-time index for each bypass independently and simultaneously, and then compared. The diastolic pressure-time index/tension-time index ratio was nearly twice as great with the vein bypass than with the internal mammary artery. This difference was further confirmed by the flow studies, in which flow through the vein ranged 2–3 times higher than internal mammary artery flow to the same coronary artery bed. Atrial pacing markedly lowered the diastolic pressure-time index/tension-time index ratio of the internal mammary artery.

Table 3. Internal mammary artery graft versus saphenous vein graft flows in humans: review of the literature

Reference	Anastomosis	IMA graft flow (ml/min)	(ml/min)	Vein graft flow	
		Range	Mean	Range	Mean
Green et al. 1968	Vein–LAD			55–100	80
	Vein–RCA			50–110	70
	IMA–LAD	10–80	50		
	IMA cut end[a]	60–260	138		
Grondin et al. 1970	Vein–RCA				52
	Vein–LAD				72
Johnson et al. 1970	All			0–185	62.5
Mitchel et al. 1970	Vein–LAD				62
	Vein–LCX				67
	Vein–RCA				72
Flemma et al. 1975	Vein–LAD			40–180	120±44
	IMA–LAD same patient	10–65	40±14		
McCormick et al. 1975	Vein–RCA/LCX			76±9	
	IMA–LAD		59±7		
Tyras et al. 1977	IMA–RCA		58±11		
	IMA cut end (right)[a]		174±76		
	IMA–LAD		65±21		
	IMA cut end (left)[a]		203±6		
Payen et al. 1986	Vein–LAD[b]				
	open chest			55–275	131±66
	closed chest			45–219	94±55
	in intensive care unit			39–421	130±120
Mean values			IMA 54±10		Veins 79±25

IMA internal mammary artery; LAD left anterior descending coronary artery; LCX left circumflex coronary artery; RCA: right coronary artery
[a] Free flow in a beaker
[b] Pulsed Doppler echocardiography with implantable microprobes
All others with electromagnetic flow probes

Blood flow and vasoactive drug effects in human internal mammary artery and saphenous vein grafts have been analyzed by McCormick et al. (1975). In the internal mammary artery–coronary artery grafts flow was 59±7 ml/min during the control period and increased to 86±9 with isoproterenol, 101±11 with phenylephrine, and 97±21 with epinephrine (**P** < 0.01 in each instance). In the aorto–coronary saphenous vein grafts, flow was 76±9 ml/min during the control period and increased to 104±14 with isoproterenol (**P** < 0.01), 102±13 with phenylephrine (**P** < 0.01), and 89±14 with epinephrine (**P** < 0.05).

As these studies were performed with the open chest, they confirm the somewhat limited flow of the internal mammary artery in comparsion to the saphenous vein during the early postoperative phase which might occasionally be inadequate (von Segesser et al. 1987b). There are several reports in the literature showing significant growth of the internal mammary arteries to match the increased demand. However, closed chest measurement of internal mammary artery blood flow in the clinical setting is difficult.

Hamby et al. (1977) have reported postoperative coronary flow measurements in two groups of randomly selected patients with either saphenous vein ($n = 27$) or internal mammary artery ($n = 25$) grafts implanted onto the left anterior descending coronary artery. Intraoperative bypass flows determined with electromagnetic flow probes were 75 ± 27 ml/min for the saphenous vein group and free flow at the cut end was 77 ± 24 ml/min for the internal mammary artery group respectively. Postoperative bypass flow was determined by Roentgen densitometry as described by Rutishauser et al. in 1967. There was no significant difference in heart rate or mean aortic pressure at the time of the flow studies. Mean graft diameters were 3.0 ± 0.5 mm for the saphenous vein group and 1.9 ± 0.3 mm for the internal mammary artery group (**P** < 0.001). The ratios of graft diameter to left anterior descending coronary artery diameter were 1.9 ± 0.3 for the saphenous vein group and 1.2 ± 0.2 for the internal mammary artery group (**P** < 0.001). The Roentgen densitometric postoperative flows were 68 ± 27 ml/min for the saphenous vein group versus 46 ± 16 ml/min for the internal mammary artery group (**P** < 0.01). The authors concluded that flow is significantly higher in saphenous vein grafts compared to internal mammary artery grafts. However, these results must be weighted by two factors: first the authors do not mention at what interval the patients were restudied, and second they do not say if any vasodilating agent was given prior to dye injection into the internal mammary artery graft which can react vigorously in contrast to saphenous vein grafts.

Payen et al. (1986) have reported flow measurements of bypass grafts with implantable microprobes for pulsed Doppler echocardiography in routine coronary artery bypass surgery. Closure of the chest altered systolic and diastolic components of flow velocity, and venous coronary bypass graft flow decreased from 131 ± 66 to 94 ± 55 ml/min (−28%; **P** < 0.01). Comparison between early postoperative values (intensive care unit) and values 6 days later showed significant increases in graft diameter from 4.2 ± 0.9 to 5.3 ± 0.9 mm (**P** < 0.01) and in graft flow from 130 ± 112 to 204 ± 86 ml/min (**P** < 0.01). Similar studies have also been performed for internal mammary artery grafts.

To study the relative flow potentials of direct internal mammary artery–coronary artery grafts and aorto–coronary artery vein grafts, Schmidt et al. (1980) measured regional myocardial perfusion at rest and following isoproterenol infusion (4–8 μg/min) in 53 patients at the time of postoperative coronary angiography. After the injection of 12 mCi of ^{133}Xe into the coronary artery or graft, washout of the radioactive xenon from the distribution of the artery or graft was measured with a multicrystal scintillation camera. Regional myocardial perfusion (ml/100g/min) was calculated with the Kety formula. A response index was used to normalize the data. The patient groups consisted of 7 normal subjects, 21 patients with vein grafts to the left anterior descending coronary artery, 16 patients with internal mammary artery grafts to the left anterior descending coronary artery, and 9 patients with internal mammary artery grafts to the marginal branch of the left circumflex coronary artery. Mean values for resting regional myocardial perfusion varied from 80 to 87 ml/100g/min. In the four groups of patients, regional myocardial perfusion following isoproterenol infusion varied from 124 to 143 ml/100g/min. The calculated response index varied from 9.6 to 14.3. The response index in patients with normal wall motion was 12.2 and the response index in 16 patients with abnormal wall motion was only 5.4. There were no significant differences between the response index of direct internal mammary artery grafts (13) or vein grafts (12.4) to an occluded left anterior descending coronary artery in patients with normal wall motion as compared to normal circulation (9.8). The data suggest that, at control coronary angiography, the internal mammary artery grafts produce the same flow response to the increased demand of isoproterenol as do vein bypasses and the normal circulation, as long as the distal bed perfused is to normal muscle.

Evaluation of postoperative flow reserve in internal mammary artery bypass grafts was performed by Johnson et al. in 1986.

A series of 24 consecutive patients with a mean proximal left anterior descending artery stenosis of 87.5% who were selected for coronary artery bypass grafting using the internal mammary artery were evaluated by exercise ^{201}Tl scintigraphy. Thallium activity, expressed as a ratio of anteroseptal activity to posterolateral wall activity (or inferior wall activity if the posterolateral was deemed abnormal), was 0.97 ± 0.15. A second group of 25 patients, with normal coronary arteries, was similarly evaluated. The mean septal to posterolateral wall thallium activity ratio for these control patients was 1.0 ± 0.15. A third group of 26 patients who underwent single-vessel percutaneous transluminal coronary angioplasty of the left anterior descending coronary artery, and a fourth group of 28 saphenous vein graft recipients were compared by stress thallium scintigraphy. ^{201}Tl activity for the vein graft group (0.96 ± 0.19) was not significantly different from that for the internal mammary artery group, whereas the flows obtained with a single attempt at angioplasty were significantly inferior (**P** < 0.05). The authors concluded that the internal mammary artery provides excellent coronary artery flow at peak myocardial demand and compares favorably to angioplasty and saphenous vein grafting. These studies confirm the clinical impression that the initially relatively low flow of the internal mammary artery–coronary artery grafts in comparison to the classical saphenous vein aortocoronary grafts finally meets the demands of the revascularized myocardium in most cases.

6.2 Expanded Use of the Internal Mammary Artery in Clinical Coronary Artery Revascularization

6.2.1 Sequential Internal Mammary Artery–Coronary Artery Anastomoses

In 1983 Kabbani et al. reported a series of eight patients who had undergone sequential bypass grafting of the internal mammary artery to the coronary arteries since 1977. The indication for this newly described procedure was either insufficient supply of adequate veins (six patients) or the presence of a diseased aortic wall (two patients). Operative procedures included left internal mammary artery bypass to the left anterior descending coronary artery and its major diagonal branch in six patients, to the obtuse marginal branch and distal left circumflex coronary artery in one patient, and two consecutive sites on the left anterior descending coronary artery in one patient. All patients became angina-free after operation for a follow-up period lasting up to 6 years. Recatheterization studies were performed in four patients, in all of whom the internal mammary arteries were found patent. The authors believed that internal mammary artery sequential grafting is an important option available to the cardiac surgeon in managing some patients with coronary artery disease.

Harjola et al. (1984) had started to perform sequential internal mammary artery-coronary artery anastomoses even earlier. This group had performed sequential double or triple left internal mammary artery bypass grafts in 61 patients with a total of 123 distal anastomoses to the left anterior descending coronary artery or its diagonal branch, between 1972 and 1983. There were 54 additional vein grafts with 102 distal anastomoses. The number of single internal mammary artery grafts in the same period of time was 400. Hospital mortality was 2 patients (3%) with a late mortality of 7 patients (11%), 2 of them being heart-related.

There were 50 patients with one or more postoperative angiograms available for analysis after a mean follow-up time of 35 (0.5–128) months. The late patency of the left internal mammary artery anastomoses was 97% (98/101) and 82% (84/102) of the vein anastomoses. There were 2 anastomotic left internal mammary artery occlusions to the left diagonal coronary artery at 2 weeks and 10 months respectively, and to the left anterior descending coronary artery at 13 months. No left internal mammary artery graft had become completely occluded. According to the trend analysis, there was a 97.5% patency at 5 years, and 95.7% at 10 years with left internal mammary artery grafts compared to 78.4% and 67.9%, respectively, with vein grafts. A total of 10 left internal mammary artery grafts were dilated, 2 narrowed, and 36 unchanged at late angiography. The authors concluded that sequential left internal mammary artery graft, in appropriate cases, seems to result in the best patency rate of all types of grafts. Further studies on sequential left internal mammary artery- coronary artery grafting were reported in 1983 by Hanna et al. (**n** = 4), in 1984 by Tector et al (**n** = 29) and in 1985 by Faidutti and von Segesser (**n** = 15), and Kamath et al. (**n** = 87).

6.2.2 Free (Aortocoronary) Internal Mammary Artery Grafts

Loop et al. (1973) described the technical feasibility of free internal mammary artery grafts in the aortocoronary artery position. In 1986 the same group reported the results of the Cleveland clinic with free internal mammary artery grafts (Loop et al. 1986b). Free internal mammary artery grafts were placed in 156 patients between 1971 and 1985. Preoperative and clinical variables were similar to those of other series of isolated coronary artery bypass grafts. Of 244 total internal mammary artery grafts, 166 were in the aortocoronary position and were performed mainly because of unsuitable saphenous veins or to gain additional graft length. One patient (0.6%) died during hospitalization. Perioperative complications included respiratory dysfunction in 16 (10.3%), reoperation for bleeding in 13 (8.0%), stroke in 4 (2.6%), myocardial infarction in 3 (1.9%), and wound complications in 2 (1.3%). Morbidity occurred significantly more often in the 1971-1975 period. Subsequently, 8 (7.0%) had reoperation (6-158 months; mean 99 months). After a 98-month mean follow-up, the 10-year actuarial survival rate including all causes of death was 73.3%. Of 40 free grafts restudied within 18 months of operation, 31 (77%) were patent. The higher rate of early occlusion is attributed to technical problems early in the authors' experience, especially construction of the aortic anastomosis. However, 32 of 35 (91%) free grafts studied after more than 18 months (mean 94 months) were open. They also reported that 50 of 58 (86%) free internal mammary artery grafts placed to the left anterior descending coronary artery, 7 of 9 (78%) to the left circumflex coronary artery, and 6 of 8 (75%) to the right coronary artery were patent. Sequential catheterization showed that, of 24 free grafts open at 9 months, 24 remained patent at 80 months; when 6 of these were restudied at 93 months (third graft catheterization) and 2 at 125 months (fourth graft catheterization), all were patent. These late studies of free internal mammary artery grafts showed no evidence of graft atherosclerosis. The authors concluded that the free internal mammary artery grafts, like the in situ internal mammary artery grafts, appeared to have relative immunity from atherosclerosis, and that these findings justify the wider use of free internal mammary artery grafts. In the meanwhile Aarnio et al. (1988) have shown that prostacyclin production in the experimental setting is similar for free and in situ internal mammary artery grafts, and this might explain, at least in part, the results of Loop et al. (1986b; see also Sect. 5.2.1.).

6.2.3 Bilateral Internal Mammary Artery-Coronary Artery Grafting

Bilateral internal mammary artery implants were already performed being by Favaloro in 1968 at the time of introduction of direct coronary artery revascularization (Favaloro 1968a). Suzuki et al. reported in 1973 a series of ten coronary artery revascularizations using both internal mammary arteries.

Barner reported in 1974 on bilateral internal mammary artery-coronary artery bypass in 100 patients with angina associated with 35 single vein grafts and four double vein grafts (period: 1972-1974) (Barner 1974a). Hospital mortality at that time was 8%. Postoperative catheterization revealed patency of 80 of 84 (95%) right internal mammary artery grafts, 82 of 84 (97%) left internal mammary artery grafts and 36 of 41 (88%) vein grafts. At 1 year, 22 of 23 (96%) right internal mammary artery grafts and 22 of 22 left internal mammary artery grafts remained patent. There were 2 late deaths, 1 late infarction, and 3 of 23 patients with angina at 1 year. Of 45 internal mammary artery grafts, 5 had diffuse narrowing. The authors concluded that the right and left internal mammary arteries were hemodynamically similar, but the right would usually not reach beyond the acute margin and was smaller than the right coronary artery one-third of the time. They further stated that the left internal mammary artery is the graft of choice for the left anterior descending coronary artery reconstruction, but use of the right internal mammary artery for right coronary artery or left anterior descending coronary artery bypass must be based on the age of the patient, the size of the coronary artery, and the distribution of atherosclerosis.

Bilateral internal mammary coronary artery grafting was also reported by Geha (1976), Jahnke and Love (1976), Loop et al. (1976), Green et al. (1979), Harjola et al. (1984), and others. In the meanwhile, technical improvements made the right internal mammary artery graft available for revascularization of the entire right coronary artery and the proximal part of the posterior descending coronary artery in most cases as well as the proximal and mid-third of the left anterior descending coronary artery (anterior crossing), the proximal part of the diagonal branch (anterior crossing), the proximal part of the left circumflex coronary artery, its proximal branches (posterior crossing through the transverse sinus), and its distal branches (posterior crossing between right pulmonary veins and inferior caval vein). More technical details are given in Sect. 7.

The question of increased surgical risk due to bilateral internal mammary artery grafting has been addressed by Cosgrove et al. in 1988 in three groups of patients who were computer-matched for recognized risk factors: year of operation, age, gender, extent of coronary artery disease, left ventricular function, completeness of myocardial revascularization, and history of congestive heart failure. The patient groups differed in that they received veins only (**n** = 338), one internal mammary artery graft (**n** = 338), or two internal mammary artery grafts (**n** = 338). The operative mortality rates for these three groups were 1.8%, 0.3%, and 0.9%, respectively (no significant difference). Analysis of perioperative morbidity showed no significant differences except for a slight increase in transfusion requirements in the group receiving two internal mammary artery grafts (**P** < 0.04). None of the patients with only vein grafts had wound complications. One patient in the group with one internal mammary artery graft had a wound complication (0.03%). Eight patients receiving two internal mammary artery grafts had wound complications (2.4%, **P** < 0.002). The prevalence of wound complications in patients with diabetes mellitus was 5.7% and in those without diabetes mellitus, 0.3% (**P** < 0.01). The prevalence of wound complications in patients less than 60 years of age was 0.2%, in patients in their 60s, 1.6%, and in patients older than 70, 3.1% (**P** < 0.01). Multivariate logistic regression analysis identified diabetes mellitus and age, but not bilateral internal mammary artery grafting as risk factors for wound complications. The authors concluded that bilateral internal mammary artery grafting did not increase surgical mortality and increased surgical morbidity by a slight increase in the transfusion requirement.

Despite the convincing figures, it has to be remembered that this study was not randomized and that for some reason, e.g., experience of the surgeon, some patients received routine saphenous vein grafts or one or two more difficult internal mammary artery grafts.

6.2.4 "Prophylactic" Coronary Artery Bypass Grafts

Elzinga and Skinner (1975) have demonstrated that a reduction of 93% of the cross sectional area of the canine circumflex coronary artery was necessary to produce a critical stenosis (degree of stenosis with minimal alteration of mean blood flow). The significance of noncritical coronary arterial stenosis (50% of its area) during cardiopulmonary bypass has been analyzed by Engelman et al. (1975) in canine experiments (**n** = 20) by injection of radioactively labeled microspheres (15 ± 5 μm). Half the animals had cardiopulmonary bypass performed at 100 mmHg perfusion pressure (pump flow rate 70–90 ml/min per kilogram body weight) and half at 50 mmHg (pump flow rate 50–70 ml/min per kilogram body weight). The study showed that the effect of a 50% coronary artery stenosis in reducing distal flow is apparent only during cardiopulmonary bypass at reduced pressure. The authors concluded that the mechanism whereby a myocardial infarction develops during cardiopulmonary bypass could evolve from the development of a "critical" stenosis out of a mild– moderate one at reduced perfusion pressure during cardiopulmonary bypass. Other studies performed since, have shown that the influence of low perfusion flow predominates over low perfusion pressure, and cardiopulmonary bypass technique has therefore evolved from "high pressure perfusion" to "high flow/low pressure perfusion".

The unpredictability of progressive coronary atherosclerosis has caused an increasing trend toward grafting arteries with less than 50% stenosis. To evaluate the patency of these grafts and the effect on the native circulation Cosgrove et al. (1981) reviewed 92 patients with 302 potentially graftable coronary arteries. Of 226 bypassed arteries, 100 had less than 50% stenosis. The mean interval between operation and catheterization was 16 months. Of the 92 patients, 45 underwent routine postoperative studies of whome 38 had symptoms and 9 had experienced a cardiac event. Patency rates were similar for grafts placed to arteries with less than 50% stenosis (79%) and to arteries with greater than 50% stenosis (81%); 40 internal mammary artery grafts had a 95% patency rate, 96.3% for those grafted to vessels with greater than 50% stenosis and 92.3% for those grafted to vessels with less than 50% stenosis. A total of 186 vein grafts had a 77.4% patency rate, 76.8% for those grafted to arteries with less than 50% stenosis and 78.2% for those grafted to arteries with greater than 50% stenosis. No difference in patency rates occurred for vein grafts to the right, circumflex, or anterior descending coronary arteries. Progressive atherosclerosis in coronary arteries was defined as an increase of at least 20% in estimated stenosis or progression to total occlusion. Progressive atherosclerosis was demonstrated in 20% of 40 nongrafted arteries with less than 50% stenosis, 63% of 100 grafted vessels with less than 50% stenosis, and 51.6% of 93 vessels with greater than 50% stenosis. Of arteries grafted with the internal mammary artery, 39% had progressive atherosclerosis and 67% of those grafted with saphenous vein (**P** < 0.05). No difference in progressive atherosclerosis was noted whether grafts were occluded (45.0%) or patent (57.5%). The authors concluded that grafts to arteries with less than 50% stenosis have patency rates similar to those with greater than 50% stenosis; internal mammary artery grafts have a higher patency rate and less progressive atherosclerosis than vein grafts to arteries with less than 50% stenosis; in arteries with less than 50% stenosis, progressive atherosclerosis is greater in grafted than in nongrafted vessels.

This is again a nonrandomized study and therefore its results can not be generalized without qualification. High flow in a minimally stenosed proximal coronary artery certainly reduces the flow rate in coronary artery grafts and low graft flow is a known cause of bypass occlusion. This appears also from the study cited above where the graft patency rates were always lower in the group with less than 50% stenosis versus the group with more than 50% stenosis, even if the differences do not reach statistical significance. However, Waller and Roberts (1980) reported that 97% of nonbypassed coronary arteries, judged to be narrowed 50% in diameter or less on preoperative coronary angiograms, were found at necropsy to be narrowed 76–100% in cross-sectional area and 3% were narrowed 51–76% in a series of 32 necropsy patients who died within 1 month of aortocoronary bypass grafting. With the confirmation of superior patency rates of internal mammary artery grafts, "prophylactic" coronary artery bypass grafting may therfore be indicated in some coronary arteries with "less than 50%" stenosis at preoperative coronary angiography.

7 Clinical Application of Internal Mammary Artery – Coronary Artery Bypass Grafting

7.1 Indications for Internal Mammary Artery–Coronary Artery Bypass Grafting

The left internal mammary artery and the aortocoronary saphenous vein graft have both been widely used as bypass grafts in treating critical stenoses of the left anterior descending coronary artery. However, there are still many surgeons who prefer the autogenous vein graft because of theoretical and practical disadvantages of the internal mammary artery which include:

1. Lower potential maximal flow through the smaller conduit that might be inadequate to prevent ischemia or infarction during times of stress (Flemma et al. 1975);
2. The more complex and time consuming procedure required to mobilize the internal mammary artery, making it less suitable in hemodynamically unstable patients and potentially depressing respiratory function (Burgess et al. 1978) and increasing the incidence of postoperative bleeding and wound complications
3. The smaller size and fragility of the internal mammary artery increases the technical difficulty in constructing the anastomosis (Lytle et al. 1980)
4. The marked response to vasoactive mediators of the internal mammary artery and the potential for spastic reactions can lead, especially in the early postoperative period, to low flow situations and eventually to low cardiac output (von Segesser et al. 1989a)

Proponents of the internal mammary artery cite in their favor:

1. High late patency rates (Grondin 1984; Okies et al. 1984; Loop et al. 1986a; Olearchyk and Magovern 1986; and others)
2. Morphological changes, including intimal hyperplasia and atherosclerotic occlusion occurring in some saphenous vein grafts placed in the arterial positions (Szilagyi et al. 1973; Spray and Roberst 1977, Bulkley and Hutchins 1977)
3. Favorable comparisons between groups with patent internal mammary artery–left anterior descending coronary artery-grafts versus aortocoronary saphenous vein–left anterior descending coronary artery grafts undergoing exercise testing (Siegel and Loop 1976, Vogel et al. 1978)
4. Elimination of the aortovenous anastomosis (Geha et al. 1975) which may cause major problems in cases with atherosclerotic plaques in the ascending aorta (Tobler and Edwards 1988)
5. The less delicate positioning of a pedicled internal mammary artery graft to avoid kinking by excessive lengthhindt

In the meanwhile the left internal mammary artery has been established as the graft with the best long-term results in revascularization of the left anterior descending coronary artery after a follow-up of more than 15 years (Cameron et al. 1986). Lefrak (1987) has reported that most cardiac surgeons performing myocardial revascularizations listed the left internal mammary artery as the graft of choice for revascularization of the left anterior descending coronary artery, and many papers on successful multiple internal mammary artery-coronary artery anastomoses (von Segesser et al. 1986a) have been published (see also Sect. 5.3).

Rankin et al. (1986) have reported on clinical and angiographic assessment of complex internal mammary artery–coronary artery bypass grafting by means of sequential, bilateral, and free internal mammary artery grafts in an effort to maximize the number of distal internal mammary artery anastomoses. Over a 15-month period, 207 patients underwent bypass graft angiography 1–32 weeks after operation. This was an 85% restudy rate for a consecutive series of coronary bypass procedures. Patency was defined as complete filling of the graft and distal vessel bypassed. A total of 841 distal vessels were grafted (4.1 per patient). The overall patency rate was 91% for 503 distal vein graft anastomoses and 99% for 338 internal mammary artery grafts. Individual patency rates of distal anastomoses, expressed as number patent/total (percentage patent), were as follows: simple vein grafts 262/285 (92%); sequential vein grafts 196/218 (90%); left internal mammary artery–left anterior descending coronary artery 109/110 (99%); left internal mammary artery–circumflex marginal artery 14/14 (100%); right internal mammary artery–right coronary artery 19/20 (95%); right internal mammary artery–left anterior descending coronary artery 10/10 (100%); right internal mammary artery–circumflex marginal artery via tranverse sinus 18/20 (90%); sequential left internal mammary artery–left anterior descending system 133/134 (99%); sequential left internal mammary artery–circumflex marginal system 15/15 (100%); free internal mammary artery 9/9 (100%); free sequential internal mammary artery 6/6 (100%). Of the 18 patent transverse sinus right internal mammary artery grafts to the circumflex marginal artery, 3 exhibited very low flow and probably were not functional.

The hospital mortality associated with internal mammary artery revascularizations was 0.4% for nonemergency and 3.1% for emergency procedures. The authors concluded that, on the basis of clinical and postoperative graft patency data, expanded use of complex internal mammary artery–coronary artery revascularization seems justified. Function of the right internal mammary artery graft to the circumflex marginal artery was suboptimal. All other complex mammary techniques had excellent patency rates as compared to vein grafts, and these differences might become even more significant in the late postoperative period. In accordance with this report, we ourselves and others have also observed some anomalies in cases with maximized use of complex internal mammary artery grafting for coronary artery revascularization, including tight internal mammary artery pedicle (see Sect. 8), inadequate flow in the early postoperative period (Sect.9), and almost impossible resuscitation if cardiac arrest occurs in patients in whom the myocardium is entirely supplied by the internal mammary arteries (Sect. 5.1.3).

On the basis of our own data and the data from the literature we recommend therefore an optimized use of the internal mammary arteries in coronary artery revascularization, including the routine use of both internal mammary arteries completed with saphenous vein grafts for all elective coronary artery revascularizations without contraindications (see Sect. 7.2).

For cases with established indications for coronary artery revascularization and three-vessel disease, this strategy results in general in a left internal mammary artery graft to the left anterior descending coronary artery or system, a right internal mammary artery graft to the right coronary artery or system and a saphenous vein graft to the left circumflex coronary artery or system and other not yet revascularized coronary arteries. Actually we tend to avoid to use only internal mammary arteries for revascularization of the entire left ventricular myocardium in order to avoid problems due to inadequate flow because of spastic reactions of the internal mammary arteries during the early postoperative period. Sequential anastomoses are performed with both internal mammary arteries and saphenous veins. However isolated end-to-side internal mammary artery anastomoses to the major coronary arteries are somewhat preferred over the sequential internal mammary artery anastomoses in order to avoid any compromise of the initially limited flow to one or both anastomosed vessels.

An optimal revascularization by the internal mammary arteries using the best grafts available for revascularization of the vessels with the greatest potential benefit from additional flow (fig. 33) in conjunction with the safest technique appears to us preferable to maximized revascularization by the internal mammary arteries. This basic concept is modified as a function of the actual anatomy, the number of vessels that have to be revascularized, and the available graft material. Complementary coronary artery en-

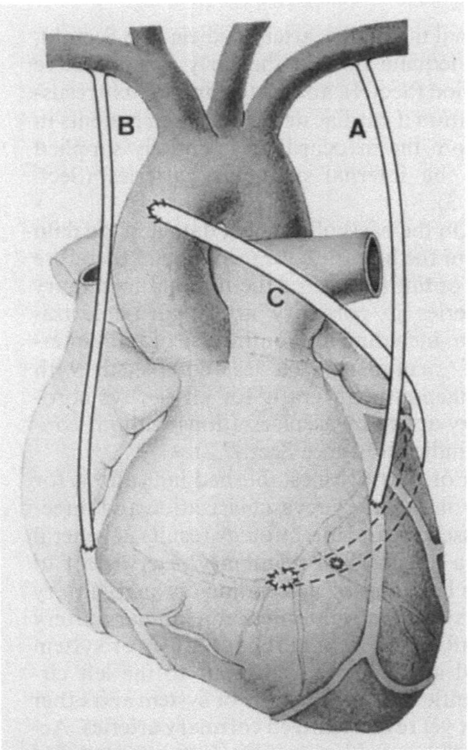

Fig. 33. Optimal coronary artery revascularization by means of bilateral internal mammary artery grafting: **A** left internal mammary artery–left anterior descending coronary artery, **B** right internal mammary artery–right coronary artery, **C** saphenous vein jump-graft to the remaining branches of the left lateral and posterior wall

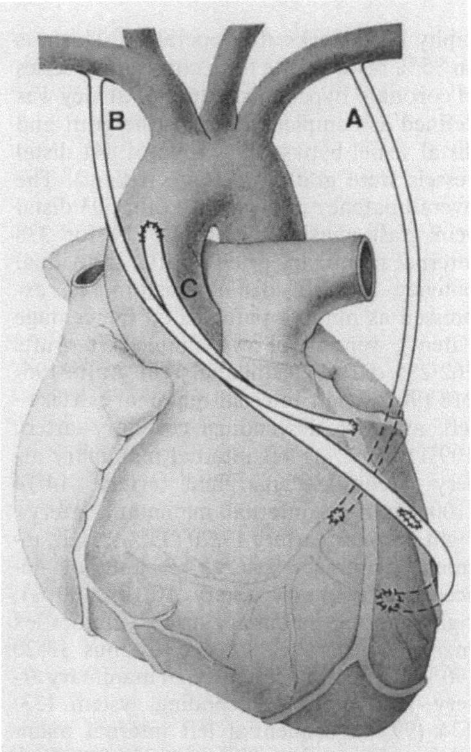

Fig. 34. Optimal coronary artery revascularization in patients with minor right coronary artery and proximal lesion of the left anterior descending coronary artery: **A** left internal mammary artery to the main branch of the proximal circumflex system, **B** right internal mammary artery to the proximal anterior descending coronary artery, **C** saphenous vein jump-graft to the remaining vessels of the lateral and posterior left ventricular wall

darterectomy and intraoperative coronary artery angioplasty are used where appropriate.

In patients with minor right coronary artery and left dominant coronary arteries both internal mammary arteries are used for revascularization of the left coronary arteries in conjunction with vein grafts. Both techniques, left internal mammary artery–circumflex coronary artery or system and right internal mammary artery–left anterior descending coronary artery or system (anterior crossing: Fig. 34) as well as right internal mammary artery–circumflex coronary artery or system (posterior crossing trough transverse sinus) and left internal mammary artery–left anterior descending coronary artery or system (Fig. 35) are applied. Retrocaval routing of the right internal mammary artery can give additional length for revascularization of relatively distal branches of the right coronary artery or the left circumflex coronary artery (Rivera et al. 1988; Williams 1989)

The internal mammary artery is given preference for revascularization of that coronary artery of the right, left anterior descending or left circumflex coronary artery system revascularizing the most functional myocardial segments.

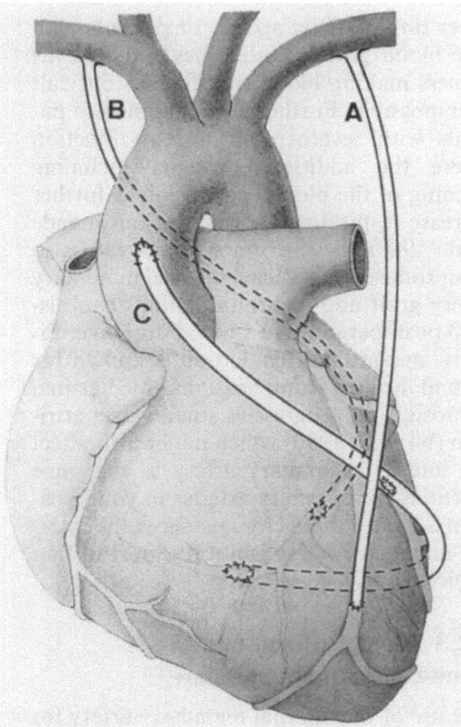

Fig. 35. Optimal coronary artery revascularization in patients with minor right coronary artery and relatively distal stenosis of the left anterior descending coronary artery: **A** left internal mammary artery to distal left anterior descending coronary artery, **B** right internal mammary artery to major branch of proximal circumflex coronary artery system, **C** saphenous vein jump-graft to the remaining vessels of the lateral and posterior left ventricular wall

7.2 Contraindications for Internal Mammary Artery–Coronary Artery Bypass Grafting

There are no absolute contraindications for internal mammary artery–coronary artery bypass grafting in patients with established indications for coronary artery revascularization, except significant internal mammary artery or subclavian artery diseases. These include atheromatous and aneurysmal lesions as well as internal mammary artery hyperplasia in coarctation of the aorta with secondary atheromatosis of the internal mammary artery and obstruction of the superior vena cava with important internal mammary artery veins.

Furthermore, with increasing experience, a number of situations have been identified where internal mammary artery–coronary artery bypass grafting was related to increased morbidity and even mortality. The observed problems are mainly due to the limited flow of internal mammary arteries in the early postoperative period, the increased intrathoracic injury because of the harvesting procedure, and the more delicate and time consuming procedure. In patients with other than coronary artery disease negative risk factors may cumulate.

7.2.1 Limited Flow in the Early Postoperative Period

Limited internal mammary artery graft flow may be inadequate to prevent ischemia or infarction during times of stress such as surgical emergency revascularization for failed percutaneous transluminal balloon angioplasty. Surgical standby during percutaneous transluminal angioplasty is still mandatory (von Segesser and Turina 1988). But the time limitations for successful revascularizations are very narrow and the ultimate goal remains reestablishment of coronary flow to the infarcted area within 60 min of acute coronary occlusion or less. During reperfusion and weaning from the pump oxygenator high, reactive, postischemic graft flows are necessary and the higher potential maximal flow through the bigger saphenous vein graft appears more appropriate. This applies also for surgical revascularization in impending infarction (Turina 1983) and acute evolving myocardial infarction (Turina and von Segesser, 1989). Furthermore aortocoronary saphenous vein grafting can be faster and technically easier to perform in the emergency setting in comparison to the more delicate and more time consuming internal mammary artery grafting. The potentially necessary high doses of vasoactive drugs during weaning from the pump oxygenator and in the early postoperative period after surgical revascularization for failed percutaneous transluminal angioplasty or evolving myocardial infarction are a further problem linked to the marked response of the internal mammary arteries to vasoactive mediators (see also Sect. 5.1.3). This applies also for complex revascularization procedures in patients with postinfarction mitral valve incompetence, postinfarction ventricular septal defect (von Segesser et al. 1989) and all other revascularization procedures in patients with severely damaged right and left ventricular ejection fraction where the potential long-term superiority of the complex internal mammary artery grafting has to be belanced against the short-term outcome with expeditious aortocoronary saphenous vein grafting.

A different segment of patients, where it appears even more evident that the internal mammary artery should be avoided for coronary artery revascularization are those who have an almost unlimited coronary artery flow prior to the actual procedure. This applies to redo coronary artery revascularizations, where sometimes old saphenous vein grafts with minor stenoses have to be replaced, to coronary artery aneurysms which have to be resected (von Segesser et al. 1987 c) and to posttraumatic coronary artery lesions. During these procedures the internal mammary artery grafts should be used for revascularization of coronary artery segments where they deliver additional blood flow or at least a similar flow to the coronary arteries. But no single internal mammary artery graft delivers immediately enough flow to the entire left coronary artery system in the absence of major collaterals. Therefore, saphenous vein grafts appear to be more indicated in reconstruction of coronary arteries after resection of proximal coronary artery aneurysms, resection of diseased old saphenous vein grafts with only minor stenoses, and proximal traumatic coronary artery injury.

7.2.2 Increased Intrathoracic Injury

Internal mammary artery bypass grafting may be contraindicated in some patients because of the increased intrathoracic injury related to the harvesting procedure. This applies to patients with major coagulation disturbances either congenital or acquired such as after antiplatelet therapy, peroral anticoagulation, failed percutaneous transluminal angioplasty (heparinization), and failed recanalization procedures (streptokinase or other thrombolytic agents) or patients with rare blood groups, antibodies and Jehovas witness making blood transfusions difficult or impossible. Furthermore it applies to patients with severe respiratory dysfunction where the additional trauma including opening of the pleural space, might further increase respiratory morbidity (Ferdinande et al. 1988). Severe emphysema can also compromise the pedicled internal mammary artery graft and pleural adhesions can disturb postoperative shed blood drainage. Finally, mediastinal irradiation is known for wound healing complications, mediastinal sclerosis, and progressive small vessel attrition (Ni et al. 1990) which might also affect the internal mammary artery to the same extent as the coronary arteries in young patients. Under these circumstances the internal mammary artery is not the graft of first choice.

7.2.3 More Difficult and Time-Consuming Procedure

The use of the internal mammary artery for coronary artery bypass grafting, which is admittedly a more delicate and time-consuming procedure, must be carefully balanced in patients with high operative risk and low benefit of longer patency rates. Relatively moderate contraindications for internal mammary artery–coronary artery grafting include: severely impaired ventricular function, complex coronary artery surgery combined with simultaneous correction of associated heart or other disease (such as valve replacements, resection of ventricular aneurysms, closure of postinfarction ventricular septal defects, surgery for arrhythmia, correction of major congenital heart disease, resection of major aneurysms of the greater vessels, and reconstructive surgery of peripheral arterial occlusive disease, very advanced age), chronic renal failure, systemic disease with or without long-term steroid treatment and other known risk factors in coronary artery revascularizations. In general it is not the isolated risk factor, but the cumulation of a number of them which should rule out the internal mammary artery or at least its expanded use for coronary artery revascularization in these patients.

7.3 Surgical Techniques of Clinical Internal Mammary Artery–Coronary Artery Bypass Grafting

7.3.1 Take-down of the Internal Mammary Arteries

The patient is positioned and prepared in the usual fashion for coronary bypass grafting, including both lower extremities. As complementary saphenous vein grafting is in most cases necessary despite expanded use of the internal mammary arteries the lower greater saphenous vein is dissected, starting from the ankle. Smaller vein segments from the area below the knee should improve velocity of flow and late patency rates (Furuse et al. 1972).

Simultaneously a midline incision is made from the suprasternal notch to halfway between the tip of the sternum and the umbilicus. By extending the incision more than usual below the xiphoid process, the lower portion of the internal mammary arteries and their continuity with the inferior epigastric arteries can be clearly visualized. The sternum is divided longitudinally, after which the left side is approached first.

At the beginning of our experience we prepared the internal mammary artery as a naked graft by means of sharp dissection with scissors and forceps. The inner thoracic wall was exposed with a rib spreader placed obliquely and kept in place by an assisting surgeon. All collaterals were ligated at their origin near the internal mammary artery with 6/0 sutures and the parietal side of the collaterals was controlled with hemoclips prior to transection. This time consuming procedure was very delicate as great care was necessary to avoid injury to the main artery, e.g., subadventitial hematomas. However, in the redo coronary artery revascularization procedure after internal mammary artery–coronary artery anastomoses, preparation of the anastomosed internal mammary artery as a naked graft might give the additional length necessary for reanastomosing the same internal mammary artery distally to the previous anastomosis.

With increasing frequency of internal mammary artery–coronary artery anastomoses the unilateral self-retaining retractor described by Favaloro in 1967 and built in our workshop was applied to elevate the sternum (Favaloro 1968 a). The pleura was opened, a longitudinal incision was made on the medial side, approximately 1 cm from the internal mammary artery with an electrobistoury and the internal mammary artery was dissected as a pedicle in association with the veins, muscle, pleura, and connective tissue. The side branches of the internal mammary artery were exposed and controlled with hemoclips and the parietal part of the collaterals was electrocoagulated.

Improved sternal retractors for internal mammary artery preparation were introduced later on. Figure 36 shows the disassembled and Fig. 37 the assembled Pilling retractor with improved handling. The main advantage of this retractor in comparison to former models is the infinitely variable angle (Fig. 38) between the vertical support and the retracting bars which can be easily adapted to the patient's chest.

A more recent retractor with various attachments is the Omnitract sternal retractor which is shown disassembled in Fig. 39 and assembled in Fig. 40. This retractor features not only an infinitely variable angle between the single vertical support and the retracting bars, but also mobile distal ends of the retracting bars (swivel rakes) which adapt spontaneously to the actual sternal curvature. Furthermore a special panel designed to prevent the lung escaping through the opened pleura during internal mammary artery preparation can be attached (Fig. 41). Other devices including hooks with an electric chain hoist have been developed and are used.

In the meanwhile retractors for internal mammary artery preparation have been designed to combine the advantages of the simple rib spreader without external support with the stable retracting angle of the retractors with external support.

Chaux and Blanche (1986) have described an internal mammary artery retractor without external support and a built-in mechanism for steadily adjustable retraction during valve surgery. This retractor has been further developed by Pilling.

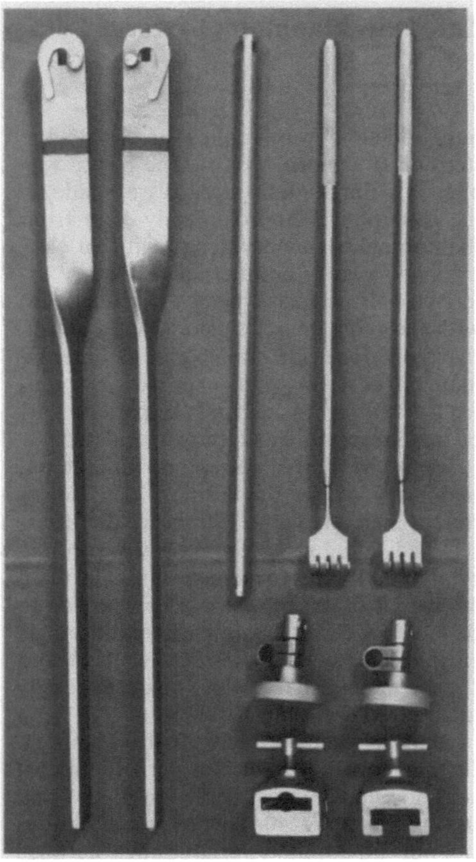

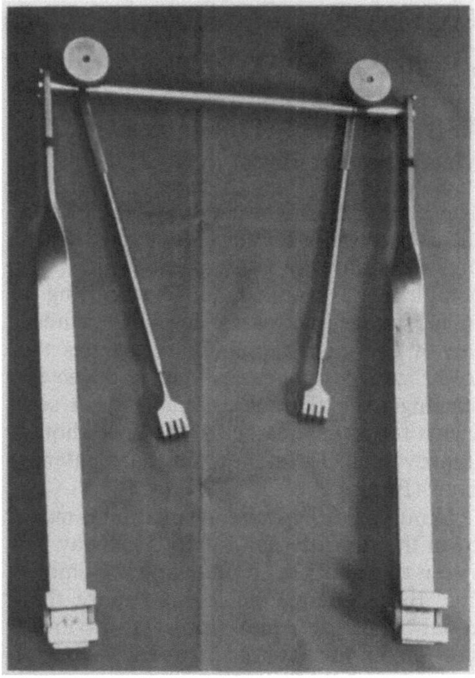

Fig. 37. Assembled Pilling sternal internal mammary artery retractor

Fig. 36. Disassembled Pilling sternal internal mammary artery retractor

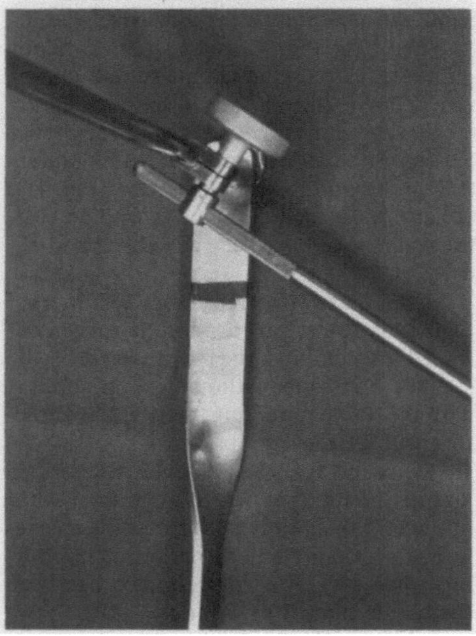

Fig. 38. Pilling sternal internal mammary artery retractor allowing infinitely variable angle between supporting bars and retracting bars

Actually we prefer the simpler Delacroix-Chevalier internal mammary artery retractor which allows anteroposterior retraction without external support. The absence of an external support is a major advantage in preparation of both internal mammary arteries where contamination can easily occur when a retractor with external support, attached to the operating table or elsewhere, is moved from the left to the right side or vice versa. The Delacroix-Chevalier internal mammary artery retractor is shown disassembled in Fig. 42. It has to be assembled either for left internal mammary artery preparation (Fig. 43: closed position; Fig. 44: open position) or for preparation of

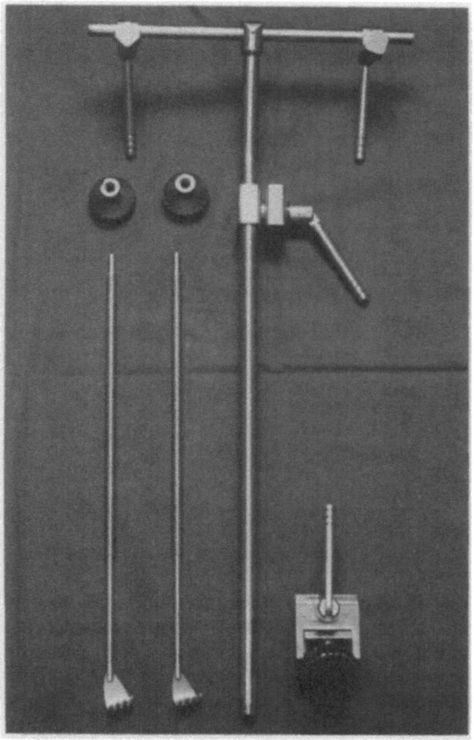

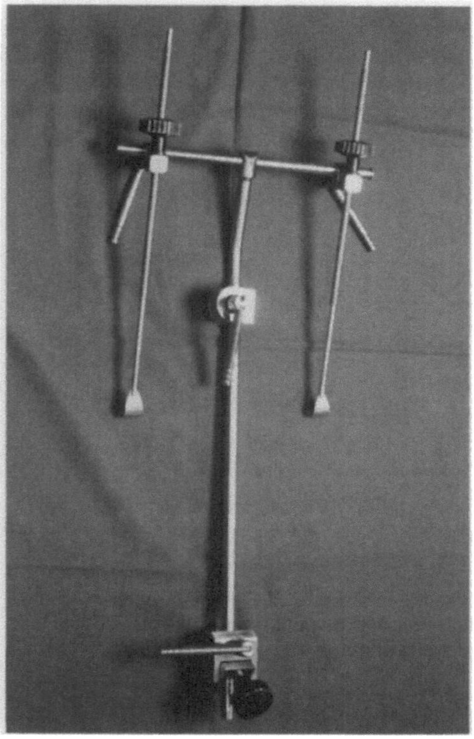

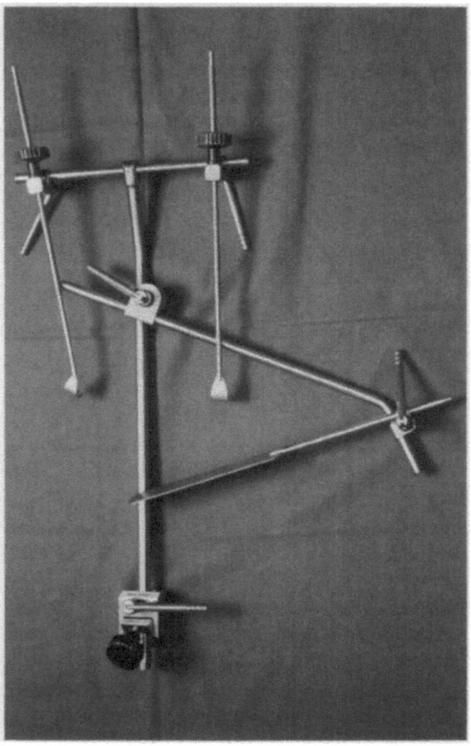

Fig. 39. Disassembled Omnitract sternal internal mammary artery retractor with single supporting bar and omniclamp that attaches to the table rail over the sterile drape

Fig. 40. Assembled Omnitract sternal internal mammary artery retractor with variable angle between single supporting bar and retracting bars on one hand and swivel rakes that align to provide better fixation on the sternum on the other

Fig. 41. Omnitract sternal internal mammary artery retractor with special malleable lung retractor panel attached

the right internal mammary artery (Fig. 45). Like the more recent retractors with external support, it features an infinitely variable angle between the supporting bar and the retracting hooks. The angle of the supporting bar in relation to the chest is given by the fixed angle between the internal supporting bar and the supporting plate resting on the contralateral sternal border. Disassembling and reassembling of the retractor from right to left or left to right internal mammary artery preparation takes less than 2 min and

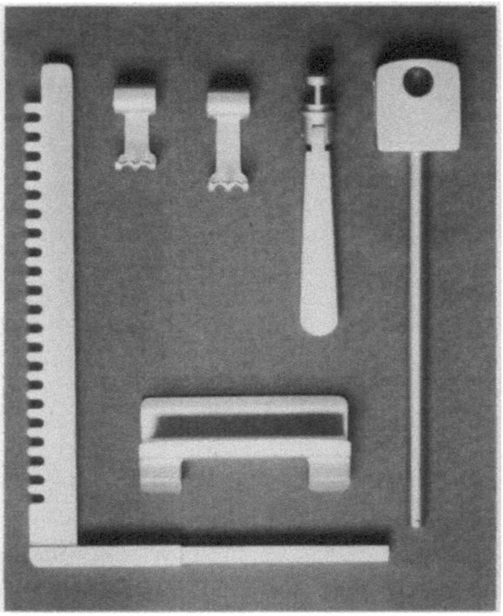

Fig. 42. Disassembled Delacroix–Chevalier sternal internal mammary artery retractor in six pieces without external support

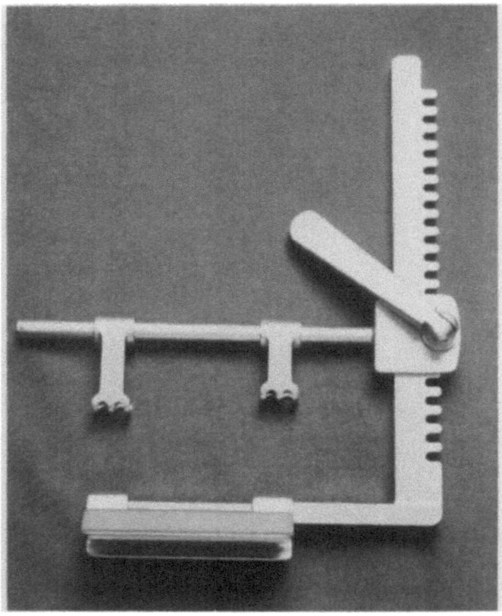

Fig. 43. Assembled Delacroix–Chevalier sternal internal mammary retractor assembled for left internal mammary artery takedown . The anteroposterior retraction is given by the fixed angle between the internal supporting bar and the supporting plate

Fig. 44. Delacroix–Chevalier sternal internal mammary retractor assembled for left internal mammary artery take-down in open position (maximum opening is 17 cm)

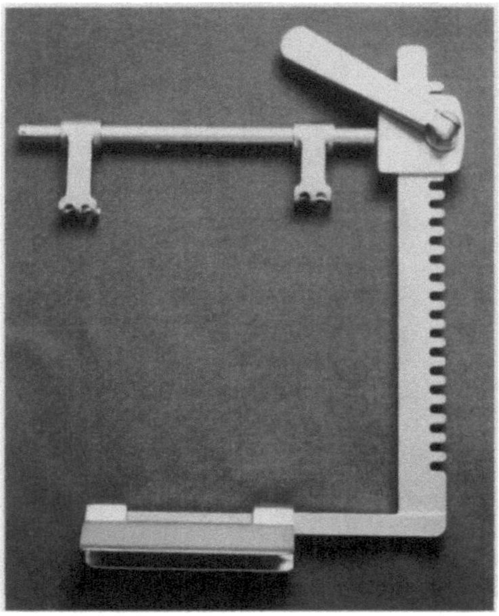

Fig. 45. Delacroix–Chevalier sternal internal mammary artery retractor assembled for right internal mammary artery take- down (the retractor is reversible in less than two minutes)

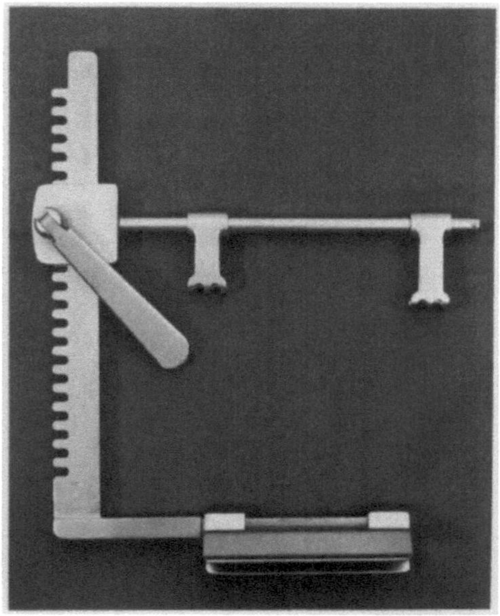

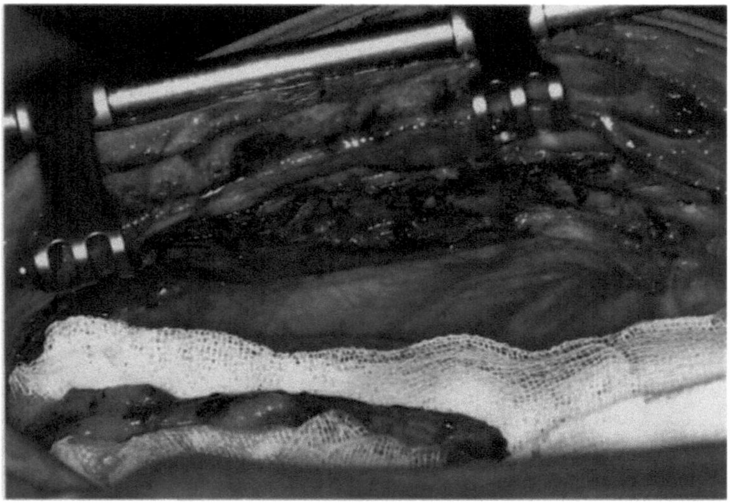

Fig. 46. The exposure of the left inner chest wall with the Delacroix–Chevalier retractor without external support is excellent

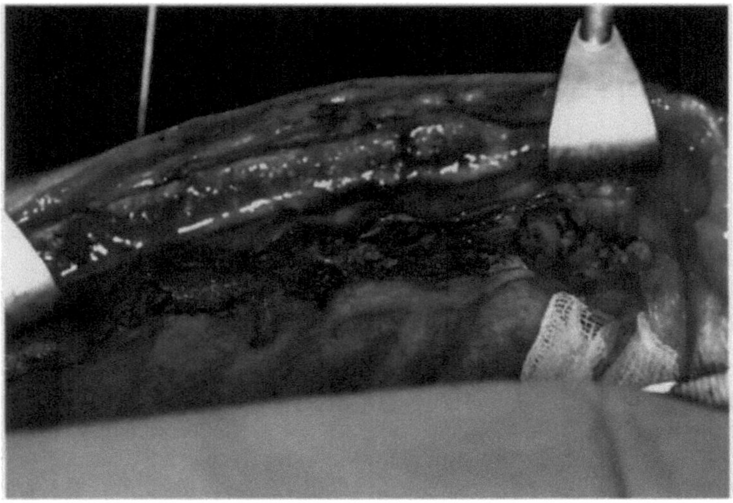

Fig. 47. The exposure of the left inner chest wall with the Omnitract retractor and external support is excellent

does not require any tools. The absence of a special lung panel has not proved to be of any disadvantage as the lung can be removed very efficiently by the anesthetist by temporary modification of the respirator parameters. For this purpose the normal ventilation rate is increased temporarily from about 12 to about 30 per minute. To compensate the increased dead space with this ventilating regimen FIO_2 is increased from 50% standard to 60% and the respiratory volume is increased by about 0.5 l/min. Adequate gas exchange during this period with modified ventilating parameters is checked by means of blood gas analyses and further adjustment is performed as appropriate. Similar approaches for temporary reduction of the lung volume have been reported by Shine et al. (1988) and Nakatsuka et al. (1989). This technique in conjunction with a well designed sternal retractor allows excellent exposure of the internal mammary artery during the take- down procedure in most cases. Figure 46 shows the exposure of the chest wall with the Delacroix–Chevalier retractor without external support in com-

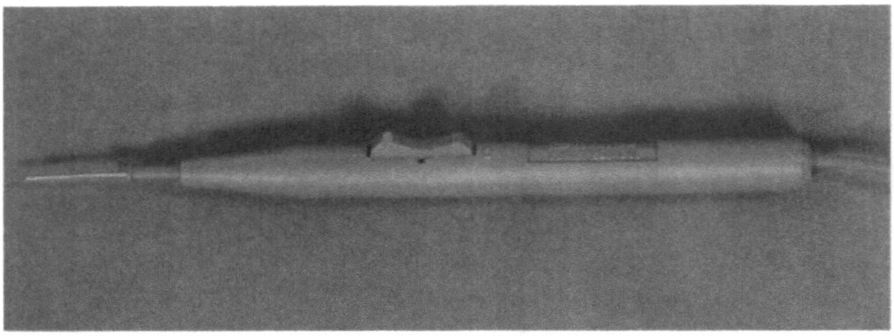

Fig. 48. Disposable and reusable light weight handle for the electrobistoury

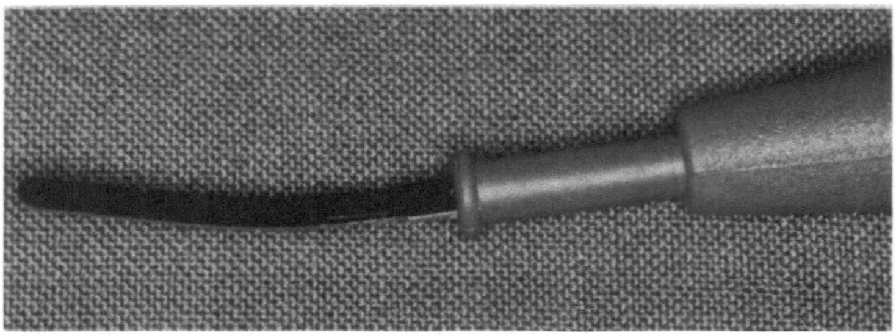

Fig. 49. Flat, rounded, and slightly bent tip for convenient internal mammary artery take-down

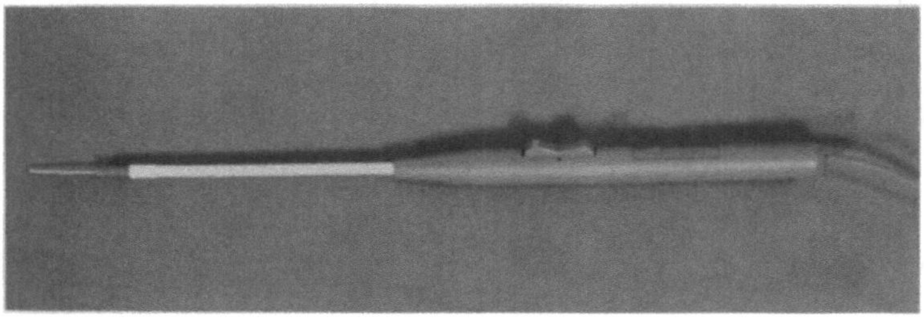

Fig. 50. Difficult sites are reached more easily with an extension that fits the handle of the electrobistoury

parison to the Omnitract retractor with external support (Fig. 47).

The actual internal mammary artery take-down procedure is performed by low power electrocautery using a disposable light-weight handle (Fig. 48) with a slightly bent flatened, rounded tip (Fig. 49) connected to a modern electronic generator (e.g. Valleylab) and coagulation current. Difficult sites are reached more easily with an extension (Fig. 50). A longitudinal incision is made on the medial and lateral side approximately 1 cm from the internal mammary artery. The artery is dissected as pedicle, including the veins, muscle, pleura, and connective tissue. The dissection begins on a cartilage, since there are no side branches of the internal mammary artery at this level. An appropriate plane can easily be found at this level and the entire pedicle can be detached between the two initial incisions. The same maneuver is repeated in sequence under two or three cartilages where best exposure can be achieved. This is in general midway between the apex and the junction of the internal mammary artery with the superior epigastric artery. The intercostal spaces are next approached and the side branches of the internal mammary artery are coagulated and transected with the electrobistoury, well away from the main internal mammary artery. By combination of manual traction with a sponge and electrocoagulation,the pedicle is separated from the underlying costal cartilages and the intercostal muscles.

Frequent cleaning of the electrocautery blade is necessary during preparation of the internal mammary artery. This can either be performed with special disposable cleaning pads (Fig. 51) or faster between the two branches of a forceps. Even better however is an efficient scrub-nurse who continually

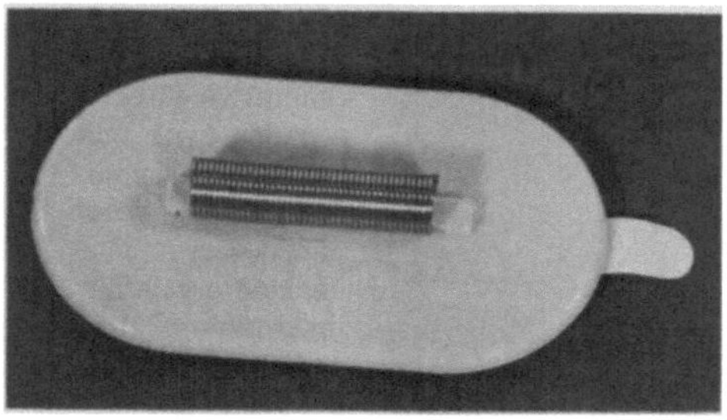

Fig. 51. Disposable cleaning pad (sticker) for the tip of the electrobistoury

replaces the used tip with a new one. The dissection is carried on cephalad to the apex of the chest. The pedicle is completely detached from the chest wall and is followed to the point of its origin at the subclavian artery. Major side branches of the internal mammary artery (see Sect. 3.2) either lateral (first intercostal artery) or medial (thymic branch) are controlled with hemoclips. To avoid internal mammary artery steal it is necessary to control all these collaterals (see also Sect. 4). Furthermore, care must be taken to avoid injury of the phrenic nerve in this region. Then the preparation is followed distally to the sixth intercostal space and if nec-

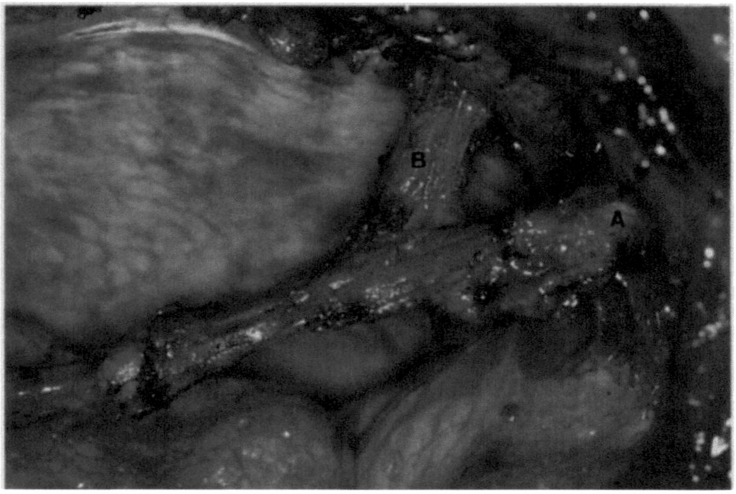

Fig. 52. Close-up view of the left internal mammary artery showing its distal bifurcation at the level of the sixth rib with: **A** the medial branch anastomosing with the superior epigastric artery and, **B** the lateral branch which follows the ribs

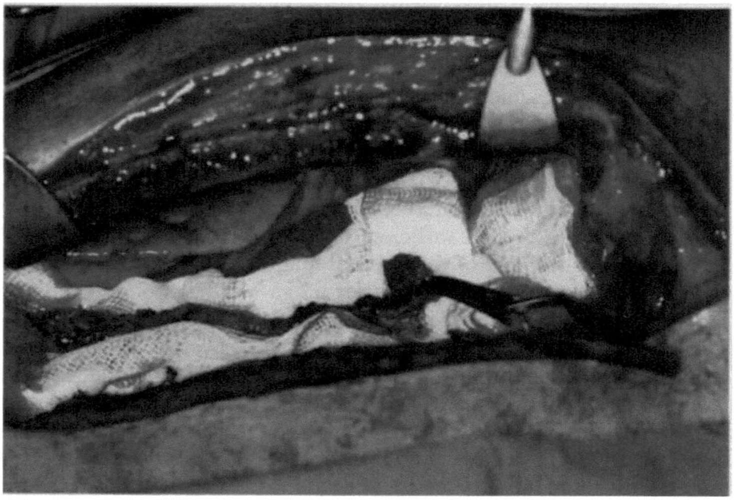

Fig. 53. Left internal mammary artery after take-down as pedicle including vein, muscle, transverse fascia, and parietal pleura

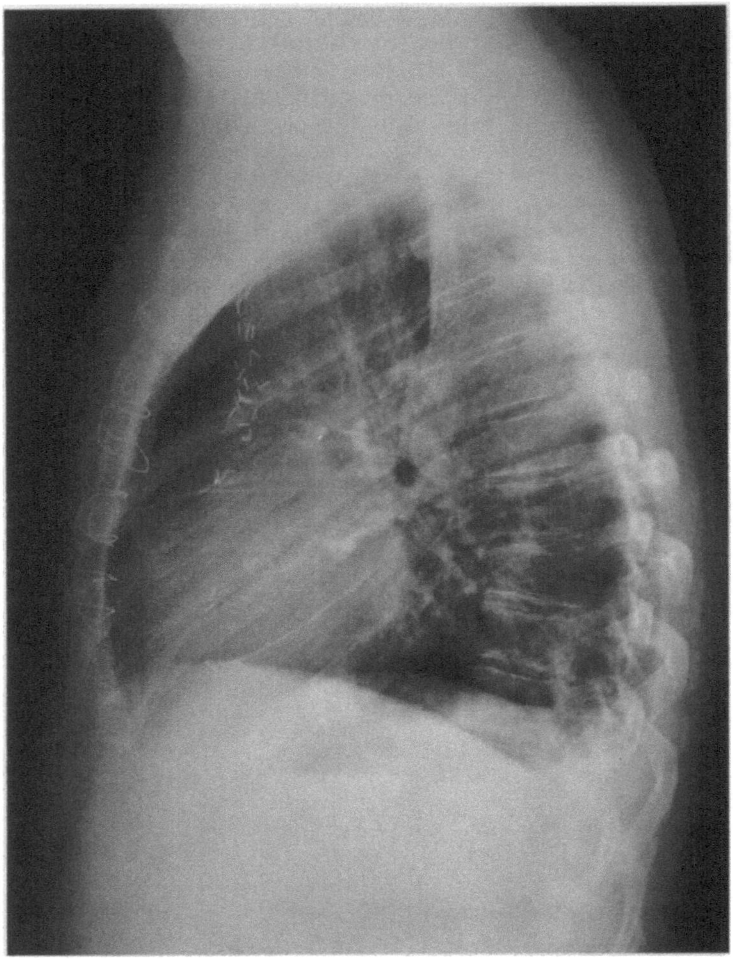

Fig. 54. Postoperative (day 7) chest X-ray (lateral view) of a patient with bilateral internal mammary artery–coronary artery anastomoses after take-down of the pedicles with multiple hemoclips

essary below to secure additional length. The rectus sheath is opened and the internal mammary artery which anastomoses at this level with the superior epigastric artery can easily be prolonged for another 5 cm. The bifurcation of the internal mammary artery at the level of the sixth intercostal space is shown in Fig. 52. When sufficient length is achieved the distal end of the internal mammary artery is secured with a clip or a ligature and the vessel is transected. Brisk bleeding of the internal mammary artery is controlled before temporary occlusion with a clip or a vascular clamp. Then the pedicle is carefully checked for possible bleeding and eventually bleeding branches are secured with hemoclips or electrocautery. Figure 53 shows the internal mammary artery pedicle after take-down, which can be performed for most cases in 10 min or less. Postoperative chest radiographs from patients with coronary artery revascularization by the means of both internal mammary arteries with and without hemoclips are shown in Figs. 54, 55 and 56.

A number of other techniques, including injection of saline prior to take-down and carbodissection (Lee 1988) have been reported. However, it remains essential to maintain adequat distance from the internal mammary artery during take-down with the electrobistoury to avoid thermal injury of the endothelium (Lehtola et al. 1989). If the preparation of the internal mammary artery

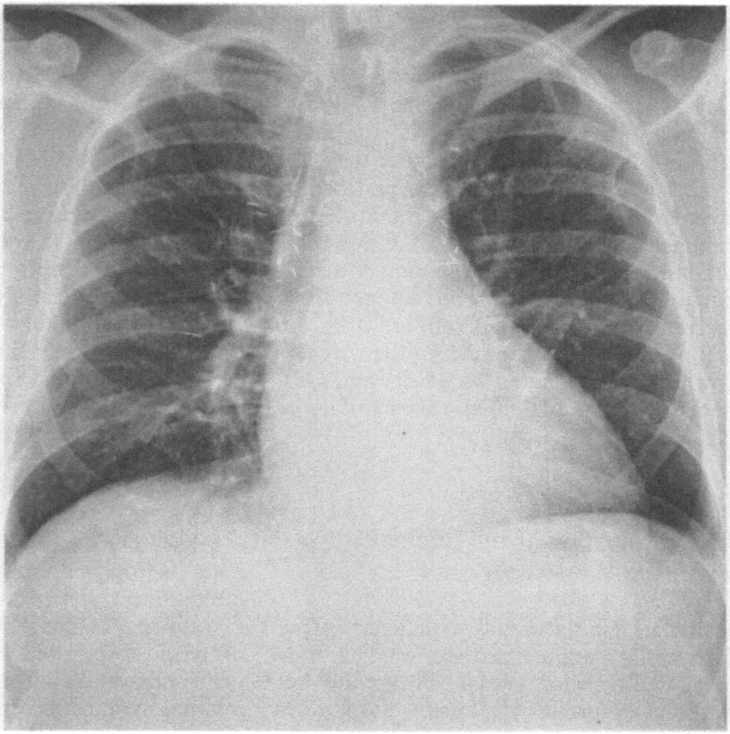

Fig. 55. Postoperative (day 7) chest X-ray (posteroanterior view) of a patient with bilateral internal mammary artery–coronary artery anastomoses after takedown of the pedicles with multiple hemoclips

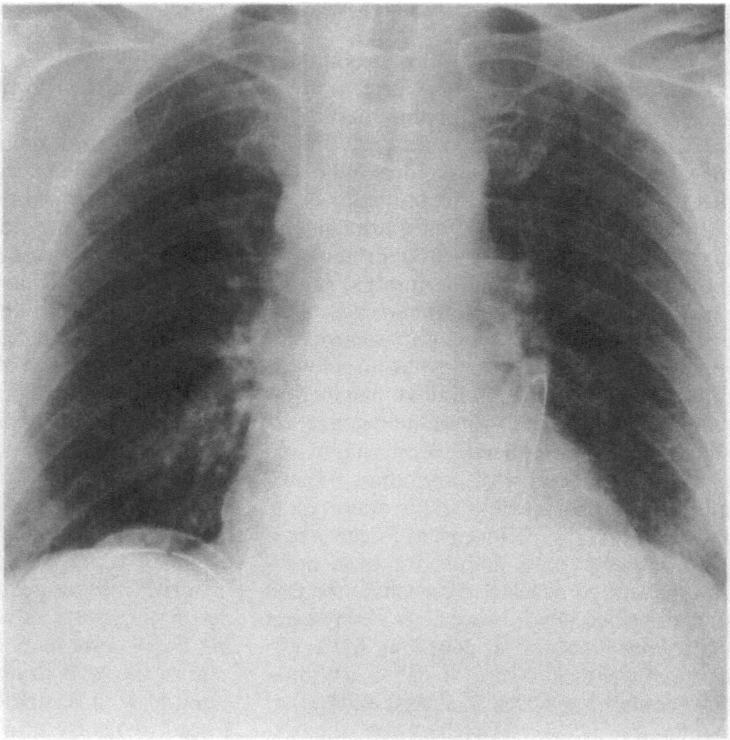

Fig. 56. Postoperative (day 2) chest X-ray (anteroposterior view) of a patient with bilateral internal mammary artery–coronary artery anastomoses after take down of the pedicles with the electrobistoury only (no hemoclips)

pedicle is well done, endothelial preservation is excellent (Lehmann et al. 1989).

After the pedicle is completely prepared it is sprayed with 1% papaverine solution, wrapped in gauze saturated with the same papaverine solution and left under the sternum. The retractor is released and transferred to the right side and the right internal mammary artery is taken down in the same fashion. Bilateral internal mammary artery preparation illlustrates the advantages of retractors without external support that can be moved on the other side by the surgeon alone without any additional help, and even more important without any failure of asepsis.

7.3.2 Evaluation of the Internal Mammary Artery

At the beginning of our experience, when the internal mammary arteries were harvested as skeletonized vessels, intramural hematomas occurred occasionally and if a hematoma was in the proximal part, the internal mammary artery had to be discarded.

With the actual preparation technique, taking the internal mammary artery down as a pedicle with surrounding tissue by means of low power electrocautery, intramural hematomas can be avoided and obvious technical errors are exceptional.

In our prior experience free internal mammary artery flow of at least 50 ml/min was required for the use of the internal mammary artery for coronary artery revascularization. If this figure was not reached, the internal mammary artery was explored with dilating probes and/or diluted papaverine solution was injected. These maneuvers resulted in general in increased internal mammary artery free flow of more than 100 ml/min. In the meanwhile, hydrostatic dilatation (Mills 1989) and special Fogarty balloon catheters with limited inflation pressure have been developed especially for this purpose (Fig. 64). However, with increasing experience it became evident that, in the absence of technical errors, so-called adequate flow could be achieved in almost all internal mammary arteries. Furthermore the exploratory and dilatatory (Green 1989) procedures have prooved to carry a substantial risk of macroscopic injury (dissection), microscopic lesions (endothelial stripping) and/or precipitation of heparin-papaverin complex. In patients with an adequate preoperative angiogram of the internal mammary arteries and brisk bleeding at transection of the pedicle the internal mammary artery flow is therefore not measured and the vessel is not explored further.

The internal mammary artery is only discarded if obvious technical errors occur during the take-down procedure, if major atherosclerotic lesions are discovered at preparation of the vessel for anastomosis, or if no flow can be achieved after exploration of a vessel without flow at the time of transection.

It has to be remembered here that in some cases witout internal mammary artery bleeding at transection of the pedicle, normal flow can be achieved by simple release of the chest spreader. In these cases, incomplete preparation of the proximal part of the internal mammary artery is most probable.

7.3.3 Cannulation, Cardiopulmonary Bypass and Cardioplegia

Simplified cardiopulmonary bypass techniques have made a significant contribution to safe and expeditious coronary artery revascularization procedures. Our preferred technique is discussed here. After opening of the pericardium, heparin is given systemically to the patient, while some pericardial stay stitches are placed. The patient's mean arterial pressure is lowered to 60 mmHg and the ascending aorta is cannulated through a single, adventitial, purse-string suture with a Sarns 24 Fr flexible aortic arch cannula as shown in Fig. 57 without any side-biting clamp. These long cannulas have the advantage that the jet occurring at the tip of all cannulas, which can mobilize atheromatous material from the aortic wall, is placed in the descending aorta rather than in the ascending aorta close to the carotid arteries. The venous blood is drained to the pump oxygenator with a single 36/51 Fr wire-reinforced two-stage or a 50 Fr single-stage re-

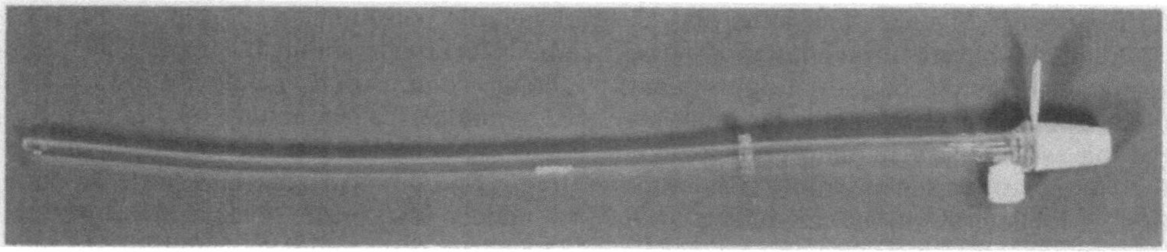

Fig. 57. 24 Fr flexible aortic arch cannula displacing the jet at the distal end of the cannula into the descending thoracic aorta. The increased resistance of the long cannula has not shown any clinically significant increase in blood trauma in comparison to the previously used shorter cannulas

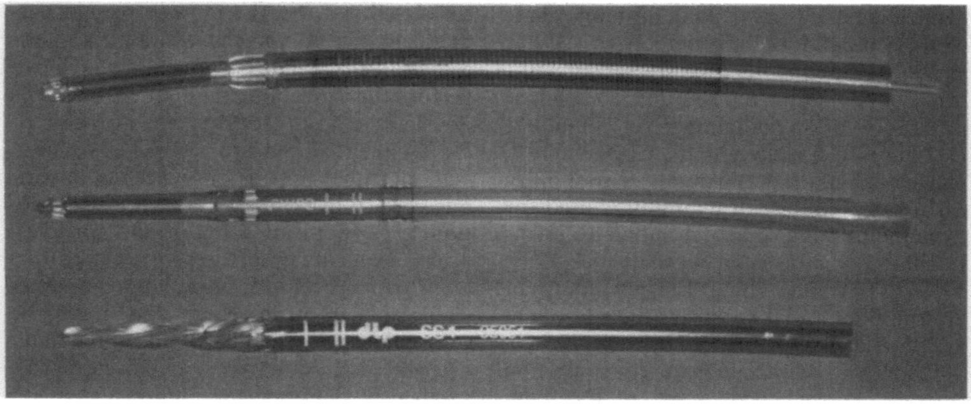

Fig. 58. State of the art venous return catheters: Top: Wire reinforced 51/36 Fr two stage cannula (Gambro). Middle: Streamlined two stage cannula with reduced outer circumference (Sarns). Below: Single stage cannula with swirl tip for improved drainage and reduced right atrial chatter (dlp)

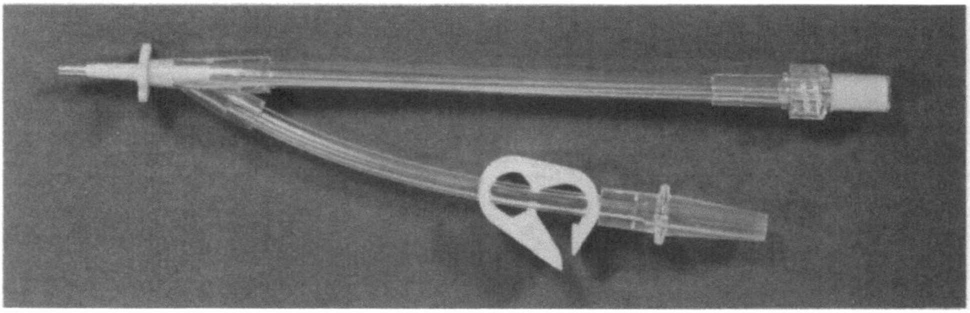

Fig. 59. Disposable cardioplegia needle combined with left venting line in a V-shape arrangement (dlp)

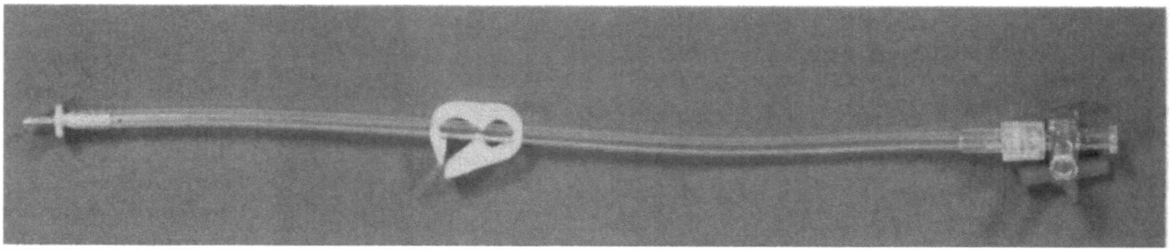

Fig. 60. Disposable cardioplegia needle with three-way stopcock for left venting (dlp)

turn catheter (Fig. 58). The latter has the advantage to reduce atrial chatter. A purse-string suture is placed at the approximate place of the single proximal anastomosis of the sole saphenous vein jump-graft required for complete revascularization in conjunction with bilateral internal mammary arteries and the combined cardioplegia needle/left vent is installed. Two samples of cardioplegia needles combined with left vents are shown in Figs. 59 and 60.

Routine cardiopulmonary bypass is performed with all crystalloid priming, complete hemodilution (hematocrit $> 20\%$) and moderate hypothermia (rectal temperature 30 °C). Between 1500 and 2000 ml of priming solution containing Na 78 mmol/l, K 2 mmol/l, Ca 0.5 mmol/l, Cl 81 mmol/l, glucose 26 g/l, and 100 mmol of sodiumbicarbonate and 20 g of mannitol is used for dynamic priming of actual bubble or membrane oxygenators (von Segesser et al. 1987, 1989, 1990) and tubing sets, including an arterial filter and if necessary the additional heat exchanger for blood cardioplegia.

In patients with left ventricular ejection fraction above 40%, cold (4 °C), high potassium cardioplegic solution is used to obtain complete standstill of the heart. Its actual composition is as follows: Na 82.5 mmol/l, K 30 mmol/l, Ca 0.5 mmol/l, Cl 113.5 mmol/l, glucose 5 g/l, mannitol 10 g/l. Sodiumbicarbonate (8.4%, 26.8 ml) is added just prior to injection. About 350 ml/m^2 of cardioplegic solution are initially injected into the aortic root to achieve complete standstill of the heart and an additional reduced dose of cardioplegic solution is given every 20 min as long as the aorta is cross-clamped. Furthermore a second cardioplegia line is connected to an automatically refilled syringe (see Fig. 61) which can perfuse the saphenous vein graft and allows excellent exposure during construction of the sequential anastomoses, or special smooth round-tipped Teflon needles of various sizes (Fig. 62) that allow selective injection of cardioplegic solution into coronary artery segments otherwise unprotected due to proximal occlusion. The latter are especially indicated for vessels that are to be revascularized with the internal mammary arteries that otherwise might never be reached by cardioplegic solution.

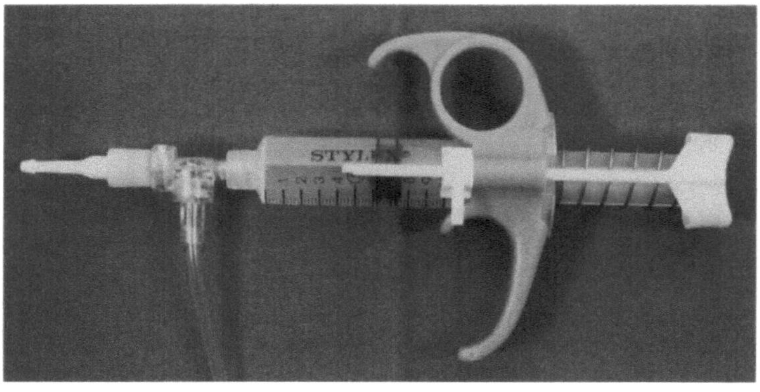

Fig. 61. Vein preparation set for convenient flushing of saphenous vein grafts during construction of sequential anastomoses and additional doses of cardioplegic solution to distal coronary artery segments (Atrium)

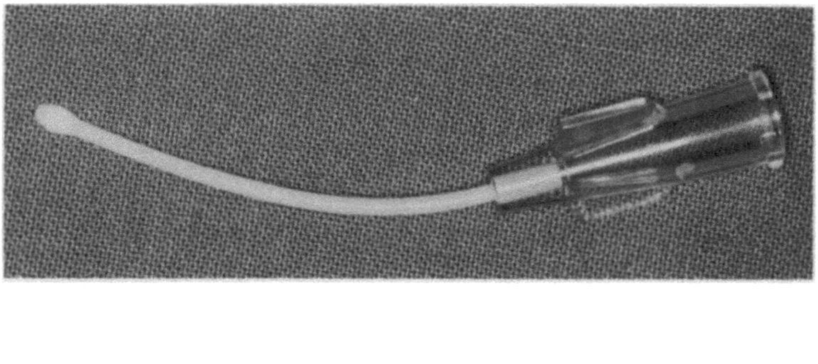

Fig. 62. Flexible, smooth, round ended Teflon needles of different sizes for selective distal intracoronary application of cardioplegic solution (dlp)

Retrograde cardioplegia through the coronary sinus (Fiore 1989) is only used if complete standstill of the heart cannot be achieved by standard anterograde cardioplegia. For this purpose we perform an additional purse-string suture on the right atrium and introduce under digital control a dlp retrograde coronary sinus perfusion cannula with flexible introducer, inflatable cuff and perfusion pressure monitoring line.

Topical hypothermia is also maintained by continuous pericardial immersion in cold saline (4 °C). The level of immersion is controlled with a drainage tube inserted into the pericardium.

Blood cardioplegia is preferred in patients with left ventricular ejection fraction below 40%. In these cases we use a double head roller-pump (Stöckert) to mix the blood coming from the pump oxygenator with the cristalloid cardioplegic solution before it goes through the additional heat exchanger to the patient. This setup allows to dose the blood/cristalloid solution ratio infinitely.

7.3.4 Internal Mammary Artery–Coronary Artery Anastomoses

After preparation of the saphenous vein, take-down of the internal mammary artery (or arteries), cannulation, and connection of the patient to the pump oxygenator, systemic cooling is initiated and cardioplegic solution is infused into the aortic root as described previously.

When complete standstill of the heart is achieved and application of the cardioplegic solution is completed the heart is inspected, including the posterior wall; the coronary arteries are identified and adequate length of the internal mammary artery pedicles is checked. For this purpose the pericardium is incised anteriorly to the phrenic nerve on both sides and the internal mammary artery pedicles are brought to the approximate location of the planned anastomoses. Saphenous vein sequential grafts are first performed in the usual fashion to the posterior and lateral walls of the heart wherever necessary. The most distal end-to-side anastomosis is performed first and the sequential side-to-side anastomoses are constructed successively. A single double-armed monofilament suture is used without fixation. In order to prevent "purse-stringing", the vein graft is irrigated with saline solution while the suture is tied with just enough force to stop major leaks. This irrigation with the vein preparation set (see Fig. 61) has the additional advantages of augmenting myocardial cooling (the graft is irrigated with cold cardioplegic solution at 4 °C), providing an estimate of runoff, flushing through micro air bubbles that may be trapped in the coronary microcirculation and permitting adequate positioning of the sequential anastomoses. The internal mammary artery–coronary artery anastomoses are performed second. A simplified set including the necessary instruments for most routine saphenous vein–and internal mammary artery–coronary artery anastomoses is depicted in Fig. 63.

7.3.4.1 End-to-Side Anastomosis Between the Internal Mammary Artery and the Coronary Arteries

The epicardium is incised over the area of coronary artery that has been selected for the anastomosis, using, e.g. a No. 15 Bard–Parker blade on the scalpel. Calcified segments of the coronary arteries should be avoided whenever possible. The anterior surface of the artery is cleared and the center of the artery is identified. The anterior wall of the artery is opened longitudinally with the scalpel so as not to damage the posterior wall. Some surgeons prefer to open the artery with a special, small, sharp-pointed scalpel or a diamond knive. The blade must enter the artery obliquely, so that it does not penetrate the posterior wall. The incison is enlarged with fine angled scissors to a length of about 3–4 mm. The epicardial incision must extend beyond each angle of the arteriotomy to facilitate the anastomosis. In cases with difficult exposure, a small myocardial spring retractor (Fig. 63) and/or coronary artery occluders (Fig. 65; Mullen et al. 1977) can be of great help. The artery is systematically sized by passing measuring probes (Figs. 66 and 67) into it, and proximal and distal patency is assessed.

The internal mammary is shortened to the appropriate length (in order to avoid limited internal mammary artery flow due to exces-

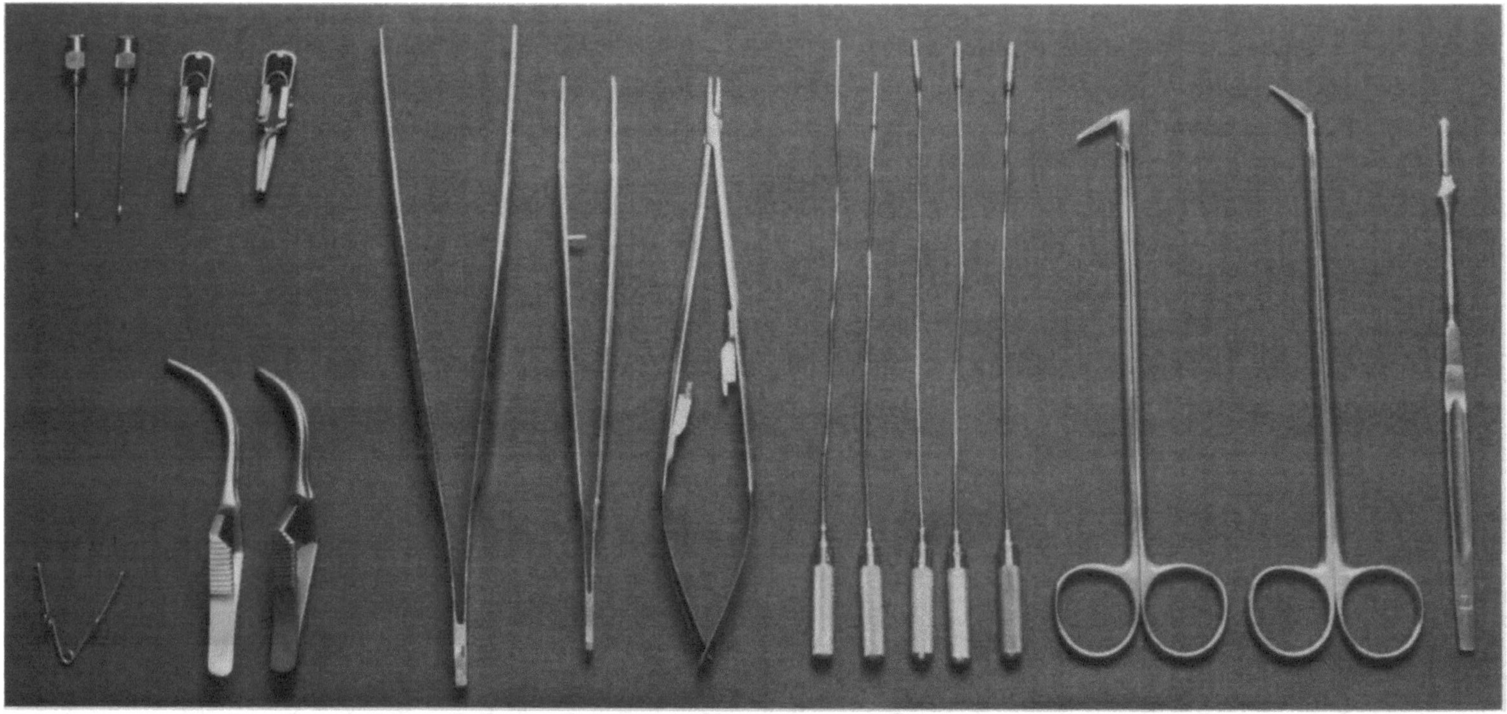

Fig. 63. Simplified surgical set including the necessary surgical instruments for expanded internal mammary artery–coronary artery grafting: **A** scalpel handle, **B** pairs of fine angled scissors (45° and 135°), **C** calibrated probes, **D** microsurgical needle holder and microsurgical forceps, **E** standard anatomical forceps, **F** large, soft vascular clamps for internal mammary artery pedicle (2), small vascular clamps for vein grafts (2), **G** fine round-tipped cannulas for internal mammary artery papaverin flush, **H** myocardial spring retractor

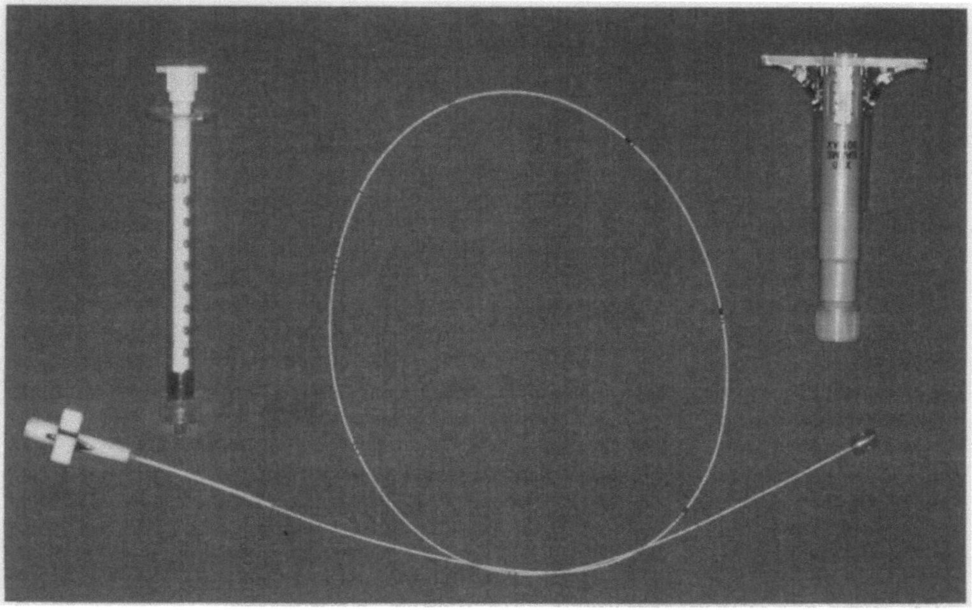

Fig. 64. Fogarty internal mammary artery graft kit for calibrated distension of the internal mammary artery after incision of the endothoracic fascia (Baxter).

sive length) and its distal end is trimmed in a "cobra-head" fashion. In cases with inadequate flow, dilatation with Parsonnet probes (Fig. 67), a special Fogarty balloon catheter (Fig. 64; Gaudiani et al. 1988) or papaverine solution can be used (see also Sect. 7.3.2). However, one has to remind, that probing of the mammary arteries damages the endothelium and impairs vasodilatation from prostacyclin and endothelium-derived relaxing factor as shown by Johns (1989).

No attempt to dissect or denude the end of the artery free from the pedicle is made (Harjola et al. 1984). For optimal anastomosis the circumference of the opening in the internal mammary artery must be slightly larger than that of the opening in the coronary artery. The end-to-side anastomosis is carried out with a single, double-armed 7/0 or 8/0 continuous monofilament polypropylene suture (e.g., Prolene 7/0, 45 cm with a BV1 Visi-Black needle or Prolene 8/0 with a BV2 Visi-Black needle) without fixation, starting at or near the inflow of the graft. Suturing can be performed either from inside both arteries (Fig. 68) and/or from

Fig. 65. Florester coronary artery occluder (Biovascular)

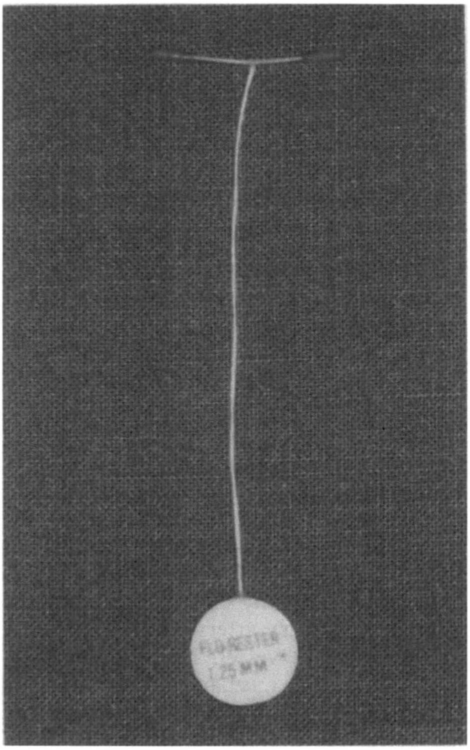

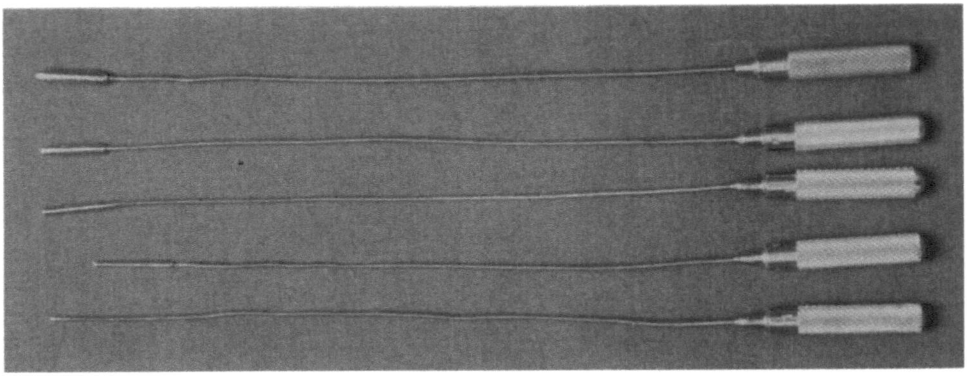

Fig. 66. Measuring metallic probes for calibration of the coronary artery and/or gentle dilatation of the internal mammary arteries

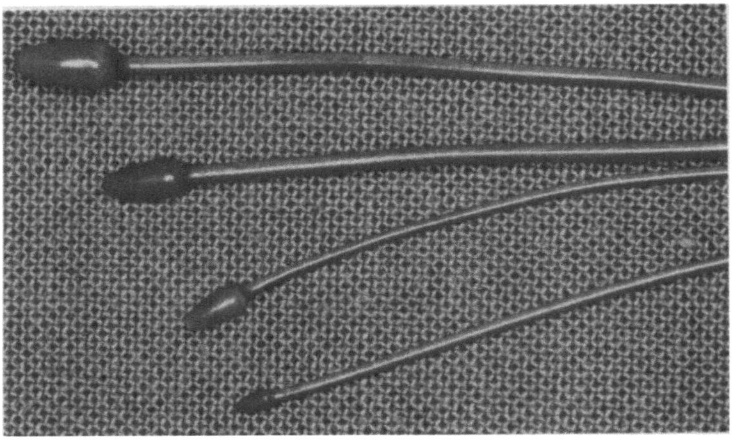

Fig. 67. Calibrated smooth plastic Parsonnet probes (Bard) for measuring the coronary arteries and/or gentle dilatation of the internal mammary arteries

outside (Fig. 69). Air is vented from the anastomotic site before the last few "bites" by temporarily opening the occluding vascular clamp. The final stitches are made in such a manner that the knot is kept away from the angle and care is taken in order to avoid "purse-stringing" when the sutures are tied. After the anastomosis is completed, the pedicle is tacked to the cardiac surface with a few stitches, to prevent any tension on the suture line or torsion due to the weight of the pedicle. Finally, the pedicle is followed through the pericardium and the passage is eventually enlarged to allow the internal mammary artery to pass smoothly to the recipient vessel. Many other techniques including mechanical anastomosing (Abe et al. 1966) have been reported in the literature. However, in our hands, the method described above provided adequate internal mammary artery–coronary artery anastomoses.

7.3.4.2 Sequential Internal Mammary Artery–Coronary Artery Grafting and Side-to-Side Anastomoses

Sequential internal mammary artery–coronary artery grafting is one important technique for expanded internal mammary artery–coronary artery revascularization. This technique can be applied with both left and right internal mammary arteries. However, the most frequent application is for revascularization of the left anterior coronary artery descending system. Some of the data show that the most distal artery of the sequential graft should be the largest artery

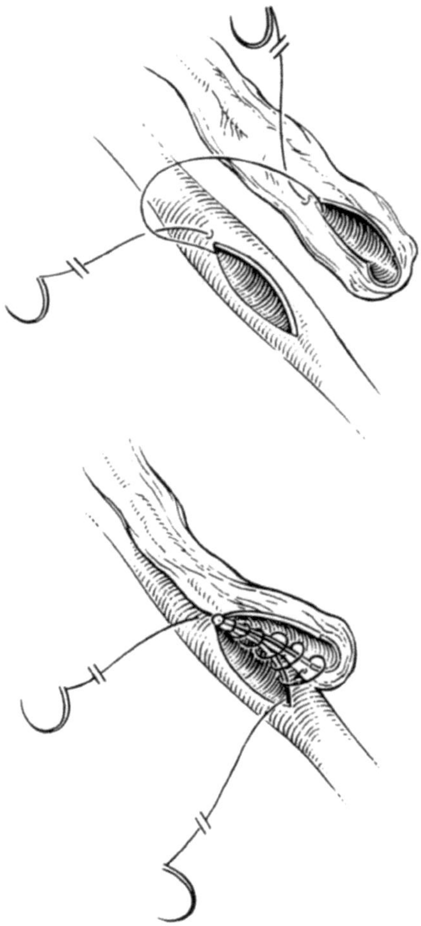

Fig. 68. Internal mammary artery–coronary artery anastomosis; suturing from inside

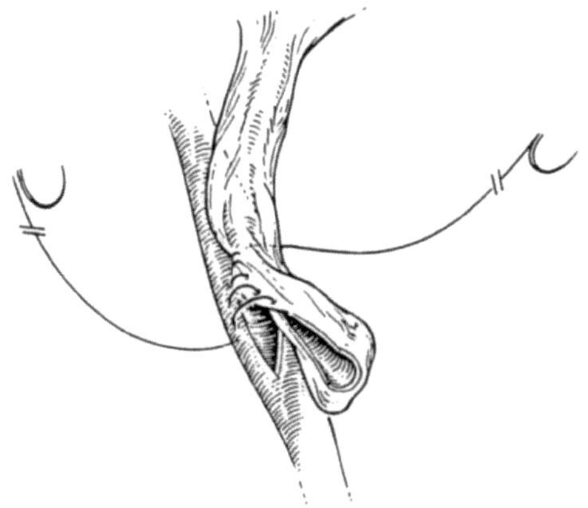

Fig. 69. Internal mammary artery–coronary artery anastomosis; suturing from outside

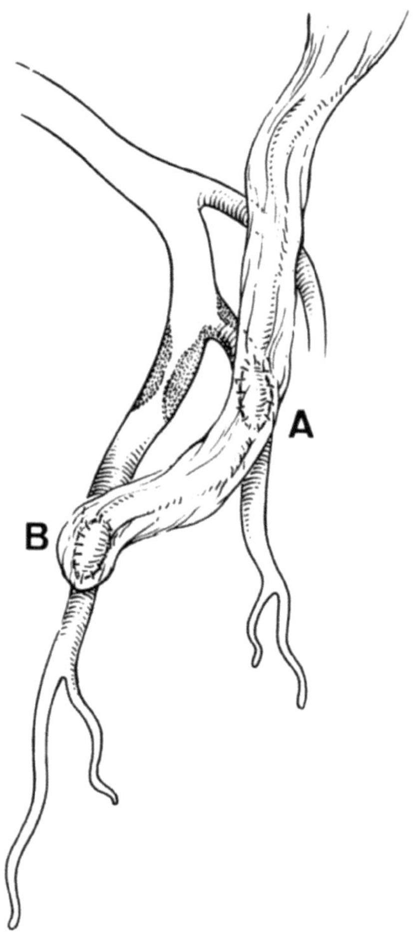

Fig. 70. Sequential left internal mammary artery anastomoses to the left anterior descending coronary artery system: **A** proximal side-to-side anastomosis to the classically minor diagonal branch, **B** distal end-to-side anastomosis to the dominant left anterior descending coronary artery

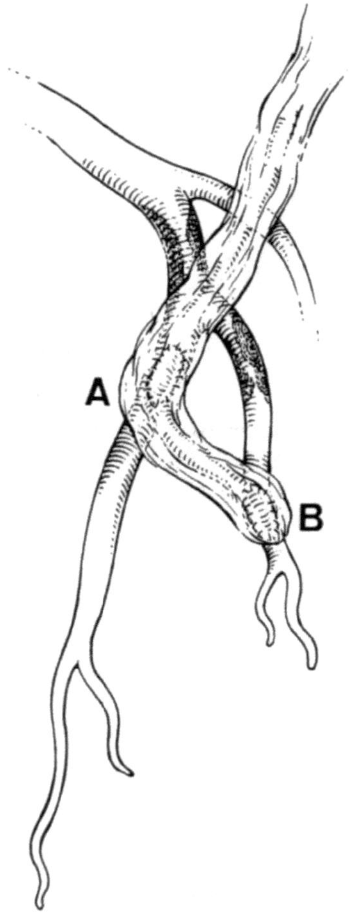

Fig. 71. Sequential internal mammary artery anastomoses to the left anterior descending coronary artery system: **A** proximal side-to-side anastomosis to the minor left anterior descending coronary artery, **B** distal end-to-side anastomosis to the dominant diagonal branch

(Reul 1985). Thus, in most cases, the diagonal branch is a side-to-side anastomosis and the anterior descending coronary artery is an end-to-side anastomosis (Fig. 70). In cases with dominant diagonal branch, severely diseased left anterior descending coronary artery, or chronic infarction in the territory of the left anterior descending coronary artery, the latter is a side-to-side anastomosis and the former is an end-to-side anastomosis (Fig. 71). In contrast to saphenous vein grafts, diamond-shaped anastomoses are more difficult to construct with the internal mammary artery. If an arteriotomy longer than the diameter of the internal mammary artery is made in the grafted artery, obstruction may result on the side of the diamond-shaped anastomosis. A small angulation of the axes between the internal mammary artery and the coronary artery may however help to align the final orientation.

The most proximal anastomoses of the internal mammary artery, i.e., the side-to-side anastomoses, are constructed first. A small (2–3 mm) coronary arteriotomy is made at the proper site at the level of the first recipient coronary vessel. The internal mammary artery is then brought to lie comfortably over the arteriotomy and the site of the corresponding incision on its posterior wall is determined. No attempt to dissect the artery free from the pedicle is made. A longitudinal incision of 8–10 mm is made on the posterior side of the pedicle and the internal mammary artery is incised for 3–4 mm. Incision of the internal mammary artery is best performed with the vessel under pressure. The anastomosis is again constructed with a continuous over-and-over suture using 7/0 or 8/0 monofilament suture material. By turning the pedicle cranially, medially, or laterally the incisions in both arteries open wide, giving an excellent view of the anastomosis (Fig. 72). As in the end-to-end anastomosis, air is vented from the anastomotic site before the last few "bites" by temporarily opening the vascular occluding clamp. With the same maneuver, patency of the distal part of the internal mammary artery can be checked.

When necessary an additional side-to-side anastomosis is performed in the same manner, a diamond-shaped anastomosis being avoided.

Then the pedicle is measured from the distal side-to-side anastomosis to the site of the final end-to-side anastomosis and shortened to adequate length. The end-to-side anastomosis is constructed as described previously (see Sect. 7.3.4.1). In some cases where kink-free construction of the distal end-to-side anastomosis appears difficult because of a wide angle between the diagonal branch and the left anterior descending coronary artery the problem may be solved either by oblique anastomoses (Fig. 73) or a final anastomosis

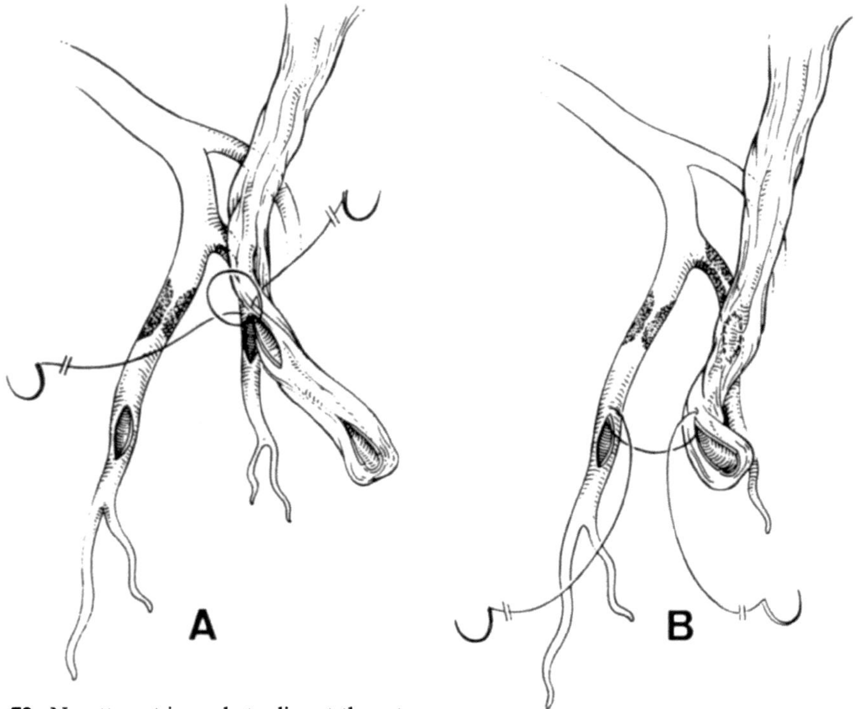

Fig. 72. No attempt is made to dissect the artery from the surrounding tissue. By turning the pedicle cranially, medially, or laterally excellent view is obtained as the incisions in both arteries open wide: **A** view of side-to-side anastomosis with intact internal mammary artery pedicle, **B** view of end-to-side anastomosis with intact pedicle

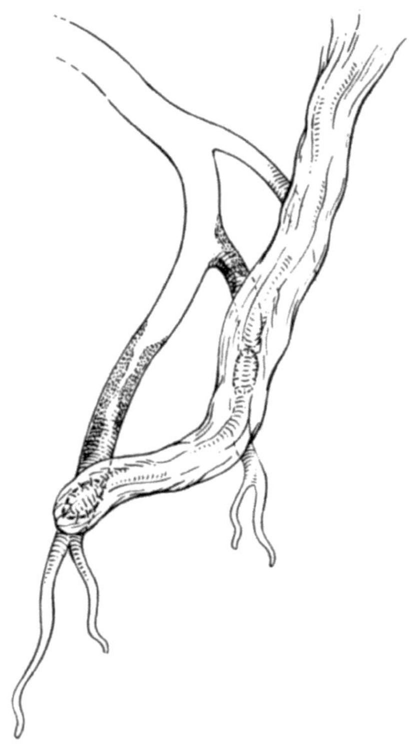

Fig. 73. Optimized path of the internal mammary artery pedicle with slightly oblique construction of the distal internal mammary artery–coronary artery anastomosis

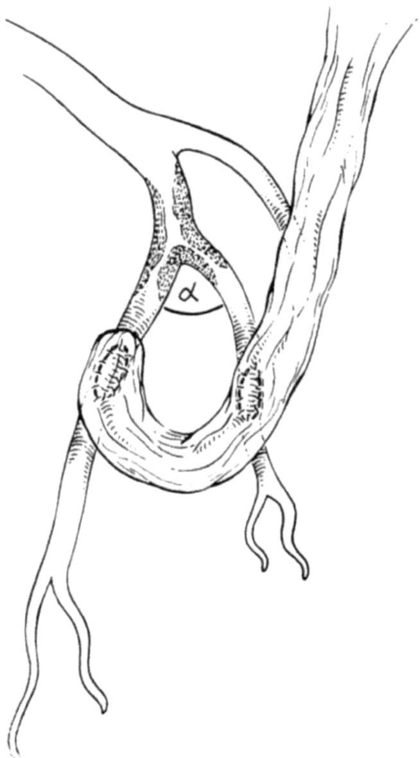

Fig. 74. In cases with wide angle (α) between the left anterior descending coronary artery and the diagonal branch, sequential internal mammary artery–coronary artery grafting can be difficult. Reversed construction of the final end-to-side anastomosis may be helpful

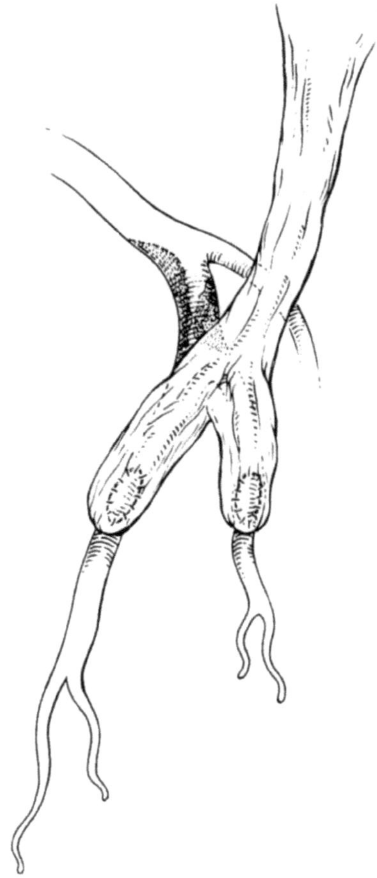

Fig. 75. Natural Y-graft constructed by using both branches of the internal mammary artery: not a routine procedure

in opposite direction (Fig. 74). However, these are suboptimal procedures that should be reserved for unforeseen problems.

7.3.4.3 Internal Mammary Artery–Coronary Artery Y-Anastomoses

In some cases with exceptionally large internal mammary arteries the two distal branches (see Fig. 52) are also of exceptional size. If one of these branches shows a diameter of 1.5 mm or more, both can be used for revascularization of the coronary arteries by construction of internal mammary artery–coronary artery Y-amastomoses. In this case the bigger internal mammary artery branch is used for revascularization of the dominant coronary artery and the smaller is used for the other coronary artery vessel to be revascularized. For this purpose a 180° twist of the internal mammary artery is acceptable in most cases, if the graft was taken down as a pedicle as the latter may serve as external support for the internal mammary artery. Proper tacking down of the pedicle is however necessary. Figure 75 shows the

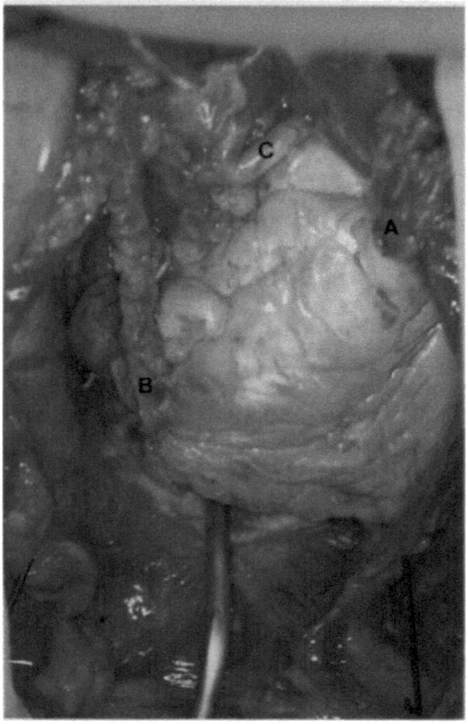

Fig. 76. Completed bilateral internal mammary artery grafts for revascularization of the left anterior descending coronary artery (**A** left internal mammary artery) and the right coronary artery (**B** right internal mammary artery) in conjunction with a vein graft (**C**) implanted onto the marginal branches

completed Y-graft after construction of the two distal end-to-side anastomoses. Like the sequential internal mammary artery–coronary artery anastomoses, internal mammary artery–coronary artery Y-anastomoses can be constructed with both left and right internal mammary arteries. The main advantage of internal mammary artery–coronary artery Y-anastomoses over sequential internal mammary artery–coronary artery anastomoses is that in the former the anastomoses cannot compromise each other. However, as the diameter of the internal mammary artery branches is in most cases below 1.5 mm this technique can not be recommended for routine use.

7.3.4.4 Bilateral Internal Mammary Artery–Coronary Artery Anastomoses

Bilateral internal mammary artery–coronary artery anastomoses are constructed similarly to the previously described unilateral internal mammary artery–coronary artery anastomoses. An intraoperative view of a case with bilateral internal mammary artery – coronary artery grafts and complementary saphenous vein jump-graft to the posterior left ventricular wall is shown in Fig. 76. End-to-side internal mammary artery–coronary artery anastomoses can be combined with side-to-side internal mam-

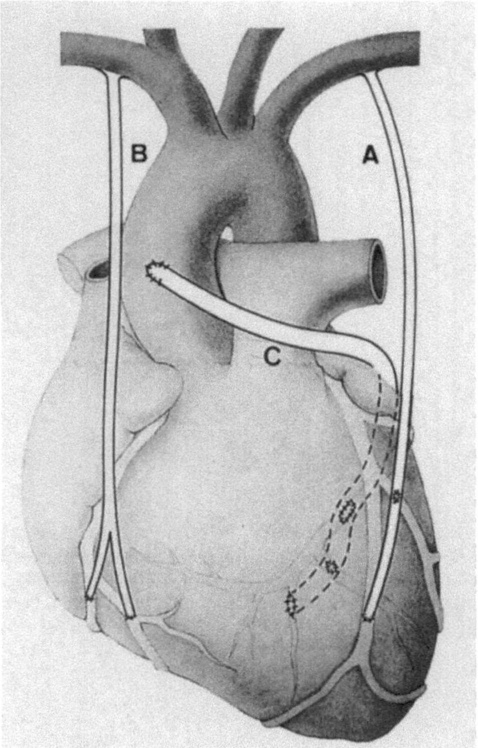

Fig. 77. Expanded internal mammary artery–coronary artery revascularization: **A** The left imternal mammary artery is used as a sequential graft for revascularization of the left anterior descending coronary artery system (diagonal branch side-to-side, left anterior descending coronary artery end-to-side), **B** the right internal mammary artery is used as a natural Y-graft with two end-to-end anastomoses (right posterior descending coronary artery and right marginal branch), **C** the left circumflex coronary artery system is revascularized by a saphenous vein jump-graft

mary artery-coronary artery anastomoses on both sides for construction of uni- or bilateral sequential and internal mammary artery Y-grafts in complex internal mammary artery grafting (Fig. 77). All sorts of combinations can be realized. In cases with inadequate length of an internal mammary artery graft for the planned revascularization procedure the internal mammary artery can be maximized in length (Sect. 7.3.4.5) or used as free graft (Sect. 7.3.4.6). This technique can allow further expansion of internal mammary coronary artery grafting.

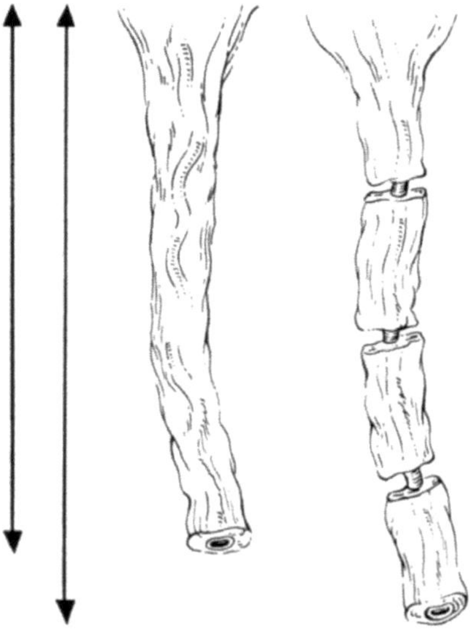

Fig. 78. Transection of the fascia and the connective tissue beneath the internal mammary artery provides additional length (modified from Cosgrove and Loop 1985)

7.3.4.5 Maximization of Internal Mammary Artery Length

The limited length of the internal mammary artery has restricted its versatility in complex internal mammary artery–coronary artery grafting. However, several technical maneuvers have evolved that maximize internal mammary artery length. Normally, the internal mammary artery takes a serpentine course along the chest wall. When dissected from the chest wall with its accompanying vein, muscle, fascia, and pleura this serpentine course of the internal mammary artery is maintained. Additional length may be obtained by multiple transverse cuts in the pleura and fascia beneath the internal mammary artery as suggested by Cosgrove and Loop (1985) and shown in Fig. 78. This maneuver allows the internal mammary artery to follow a straight course and provides additional length. Each fasciotomy made, may add as much as 1 cm length.

Proximally the internal mammary artery pedicle may be restrained by lateral pleural and thymic attachments (Cosgrove and Loop 1985). Lysis of these fibers provides additional length (Fig. 79). Furthermore, the right internal mammary vein communicates directly with the azygos system. Dividing this communication can further increase the internal mammary artery length.

An optimal path for the internal mammary artery pedicle is created either by a deep notch in the pericardium or by a craniocaudal incision anterior to the phrenic nerve. The latter can very often be performed in the pericardial zone which is free from pericardial fat and provides the most

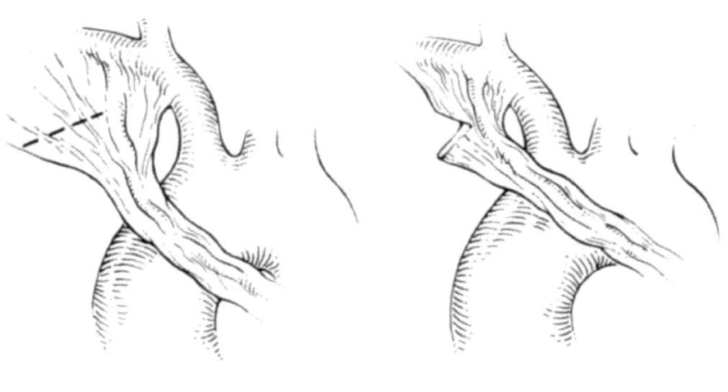

Fig. 79. Lysis of lateral pleural fibers and medial internal mammary vein increases the mobility and the usable length of the internal mammary artery (modified from Cosgrove and Loop 1985)

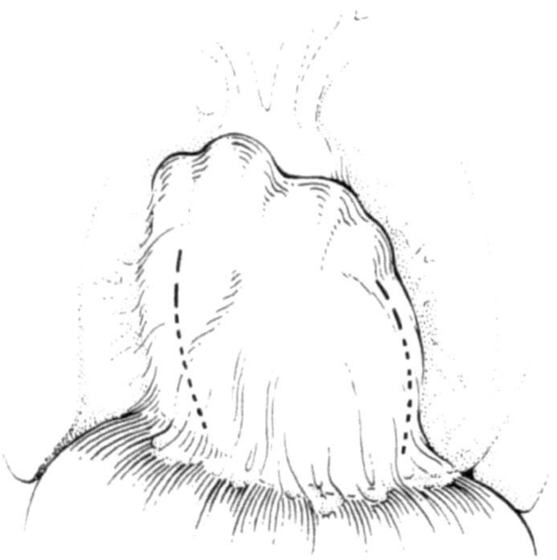

Fig. 80. Bilateral cranio-caudal incisions avoiding the phrenic nerves provide the most direct and shortest course to the coronary arteries

direct and shortest course to the heart (Fig. 80). The incision can be enlarged later on to adapt the internal mammary artery course to the beating heart and the expanding lungs. Different types of pericardial incisions have been suggested by Fledge (1987), Vander Salm (1989) and others. As mentioned before, the left circumflex coronary artery system can be reached by the right internal mammary artery through the transverse sinus. When this type of revascularization is selected the right internal mammary artery length might be rather tight during construction of the anastomoses to the circumflex coronary artery system. However, once the heart is released, there is in general adequate pedicle length available. The situation is different when the left circumflex coronary artery system is revascularized with the left internal mammary artery where the pedicle length finally required exceeds the minimal length necessary for construction of the anastomoses. The transpericardial, retrocaval route (Rivera 1988, Williams 1989) can help to reach distal branches of the right coronary artery system or the left circumflex coronary artery system with the right internal mammary artery.

Internal mammary artery–coronary artery anastomotic tension can be reduced in some cases by suturing the pericardium or a pericardial flap to the chest wall (Todd et al. 1988, Starr and Moore 1989). Other authors promoted for the internal mammary artery pedicle an initial path between parietal pleura and pericardium (Galbut et al. 1985, Martinez et al. 1988). The latter technique has the advantage that the pleura can be left intact and reduced respiratory morbidity can be expected. If internal mammary artery–coronary artery anastomotic tension cannot be eliminated by these measures, the internal mammary artery graft has to be transected at it's origin and reimplanted into the ascending aorta resulting in a free internal mammary artery graft.

7.3.4.6 Free (Aortocoronary) Internal Mammary Artery Graft Anastomoses

There are three main indications for the use of free aortocoronary internal mammary artery grafts:

1. Inadequate length of the in situ internal mammary artery for revascularization of distal coronary artery segments or construction of multiple internal mammary artery–coronary artery anastomoses. In fact, stretching the internal mammary artery pedicle may compromise an otherwise perfect complex revascularization procedure, because of angulation or stenosis at an internal mammary artery–coronary artery anastomosis
2. Avoidance of crossing the midline anterior to the heart with the right internal mammary artery for revascularization of the left anterior descending coronary artery system. In patients with reasonable probability of reoperation the in situ right internal mammary artery should not be used for this type of revascularization procedure because of the major risk of injuring or dividing the crossing internal mammary artery during reentry. The free graft will reach almost any coronary artery branch
3. An accidentally, proximally damaged internal mammary artery graft might be more easily converted into a free internal mammary artery graft with proper anastomoses than repaired by delicate microsurgical techniques in the apex of the chest

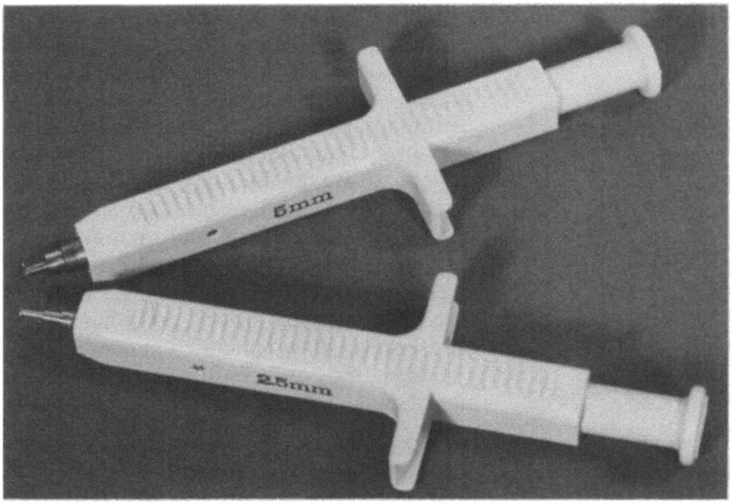

Fig. 81. Special smaller size aortic punch for direct implantation of the internal mammary artery into the ascending aorta (2.5 mm) in comparison to standard punch for saphenous vein implantation (5 mm) (Johnson & Johnson).

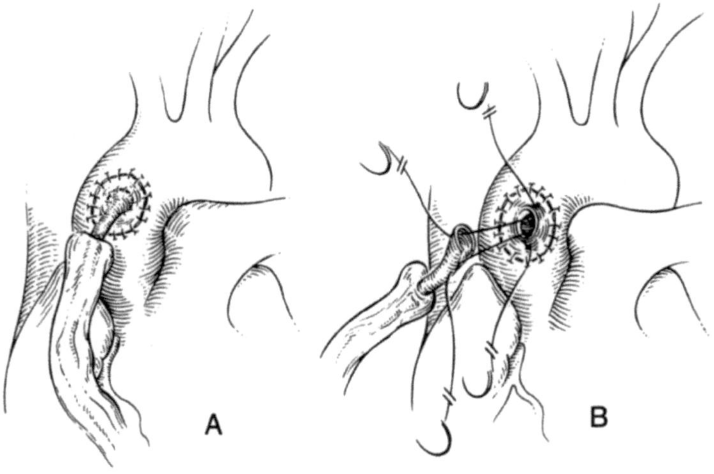

Fig. 82. Saphenous vein patch for indirect implantation of the free (aortocoronary) internal mammary artery into the ascending aorta: **A** vein patch with punched hole, **B** vein patch with suitable side branch (venous valves should be avoided)

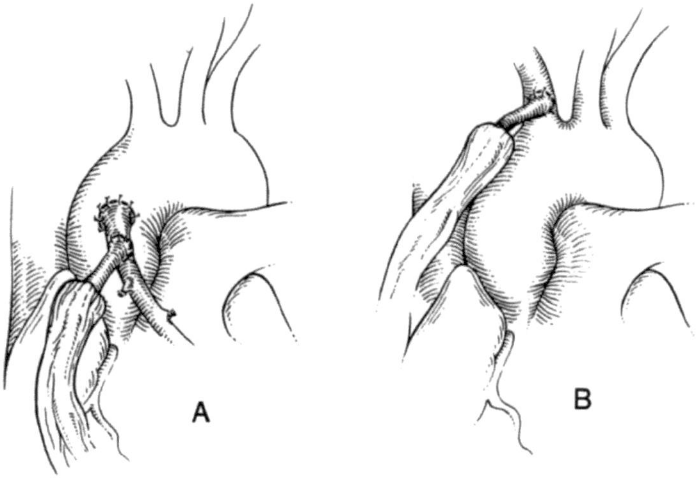

Fig. 83. Other techniques for proximal anastomoses of free (aortocoronary) internal mammary artery grafts: **A** implantation onto the hood of a saphenous vein graft, **B** implantation onto the brachiocephalic trunk

Free (aortocoronary) internal mammary artery grafts are relatively protected from atherosclerosis as shown in Sect. 6.2.2. The distal anastomoses of the free internal mammary artery graft are constructed in the same way as described for the in situ internal mammary artery graft. However, the proximal anastomosis between internal mammary artery and ascending aorta is more delicate. In the series of Loop et al. (1986b) all proximal anastomoses were constructed directly into the aorta. Special, smaller size, aortic punches are available for this purpose (Fig. 81). Other techniques include the use of a patch of saphenous vein or autologous pericardium (Kanter and Barner 1987) with a punched hole, a patch of saphenous vein containing a suitable side branch as suggested by Schimert et al. (1975) and shown in Fig. 82 or implantation onto the hood of a saphenous vein graft (Barner 1973), onto the hood of an in situ internal mammary artery graft (Sauvage et al. 1986), or implantation onto the brachiocephalic trunk as shown in Fig. 83.

7.3.5 Weaning from Cardiopulmonary Bypass

During construction of the last distal anastomosis, rewarming of the patient with the pump oxygenator is started. If complex multiple internal mammary artery–coronary artery grafting has been performed, there will be only a short time available for rewarming as in situ internal mammary artery grafts do not need proximal anastomoses. In most routine cases with bilateral internal mammary grafts, only one venous sequential graft will have to be implanted onto the ascending aorta. At completion of the last internal mammary artery–coronary artery anastomosis, warm cardioplegic solution is given, the occluding vascular clamps are removed from both internal mammary artery pedicles, the ascending aorta is released, and the tightness of the distal anastomoses is checked. An additional stitch is much easier to place with the heart standing still or fibrillating in comparison to the heart beating. Medicamentous or, if necessary, electrical defibrillation of the heart is achieved while the proximal anastomoses are constructed and temporary pacing wires are installed. There can be no doubt that the reduced number of proximal anastomoses resulting from expanded in situ internal mammary artery grafting allows one to recover most of the additional time that is necessary for take-down of the internal mammary arteries. After adequate rewarming (rectal temperature > 35 °C), sufficient reperfusion of the heart (at least 10 min after release of the aortic clamp) and control of blood gases, weaning from cardiopulmonary bypass is started. Circumspect filling of the four cavities of the heart, to achieve maximal benefit by Starling's mechanism, is of prime importance in this critical phase. Small doses of positive inotropic drugs and Ca^{++} are given as bolus, during reduction of pump flow, when necessary, to achieve adequate hemodynamics. A continuous, low dose infusion of nitrates and/or nifedipin to prevent from internal mammary artery spasm has been advocated, for patients receiving single and multiple internal mammary artery grafts, throughout the procedure, i.e., during harvesting, cardioplegic standstill of the heart, rewarming, reperfusion, weaning from cardiopulmonary bypass, and the early postoperative phase in the intensive care unit, where it is replaced with peroral anticalcic drugs when the patient is stable. Bradycardia is corrected with atrial, ventricular, or sequential pacing as appropriate. After stabilization in an isovolemic state the cannulas are withdrawn and heparin is reversed with protamine as usual. Continuous visual checks of cardiac contractility and volemia are necessary in this critical period, where eventually occurring low cardiac output must be recognized and treated quickly. As reported previously (see Sect. 5.1.3.), pharmacological interventions are difficult when a low cardiac output state has occurred as they can provoke adverse spastic reactions of the internal mammary arteries with consequently reduced perfusion of the grafted coronary arteries leading to a vicious circle.

7.3.6 Hemostasis

Thorough hemostasis of all parts of the operating field is necessary in internal mammary artery–coronary artery grafting to reduce the incidence of postoperative bleeding complications due to the increased intrathoracic injury. This includes the graft anastomoses, the cannulation sites, the bed of the prepared internal mammary artery on the inner thoracic wall, the site of transection at the level of the superior epigastric artery, the transected major internal mammary artery and vein branches at the apex of the chest, the internal mammary artery pedicles, the mobilized thymus, the pericardial incisions, the sternal borders, and the region of the suprasternal notch. Local application of hemostatic agents such as collagen sponges or fibrin glue can help to control eventual bleeding from the internal mammary artery bed.

Cardiopulmonary bypass with nonhemic priming medium, acceptance of normovolemic anemia, use of nonhemic volume expanders, and further blood salvaging techniques have been developed including autotransfusion and hemofiltration (Sect. 7.3.6.1), preservation and/or reactivation of platelets and coagulation factors (Sect. 7.3.6.2) and improved cardiopulmonary bypass equipment (Sect. 7.3.6.3).

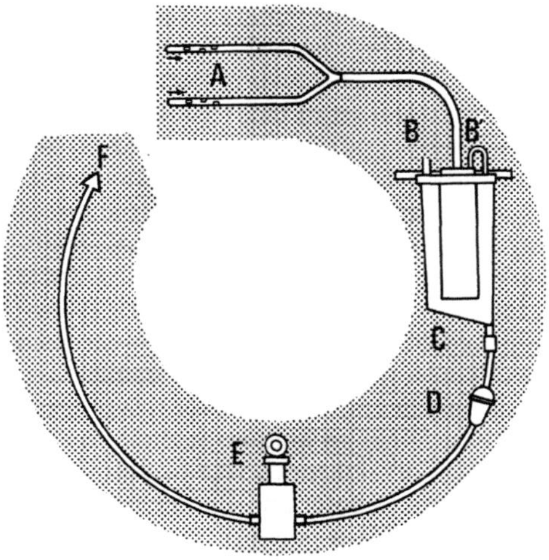

Fig. 84. Mediastinal shed blood autotransfusion system including: **A** chest tubes, **B** wall suction, **B'** shunt permitting drainage in case of clotted cardiotomy filter, **C** heparinized cardiotomy reservoir, **D** filter, **E** volumetric pump with **F** venous infusion line

7.3.6.1 Autotransfusion

Transfusion of oxygenator sump blood, centrifuged or uncentrifuged, and retransfusion of mediastinal shed blood, collected with the cardiotomy reservoir and retransfused with a volumetric pump (Fig. 84) are widely used. Retransfusion of processed red cells concentrated with a programmable cell saver (von Segesser et al. 1986) is more expensive, but allows recovery of substantial amounts of concentrated red cells. It appears especially indicated in cases with expected significant blood loss or lack of bank blood. Hemofiltration (Boldt et al. 1989, von Segesser et al. 1990 b) is an other approach allowing not only salvage of red cells but also platelets and plasma. Each method has its specific advantages and disadvantages. Transfusion of oxygenator sump blood is cheap, but limited in amount and the transfusate is heparinized. Postoperative retransfusion of mediastinal shed blood collected with the cardiotomy reservoir after neutralization of heparin delivers larger amounts but implies transfusion of defibrinated blood with fibrin split products and free plasma hemoglobin (Hartz et al. 1988). Cell savers separate the aspirated blood into plasma and detritus which are discarded during the washing process, and red cells which are resuspended in saline without quantitative limitation. The transfusate is concentrated with a hematocrit of up to 60% and has low heparin content (< 1000 U/l). Platelets and coagulation factors are lost however. Improved devices, using plasma filtration techniques for recovery of red cells, platelets, and plasma are actually under development.

7.3.6.2 Preservation and/or Reactivation of Platelets and Coagulation Factors

Preservation of platelets and coagulation factors can be performed by withdrawal of whole blood immediately before cardiopulmonary bypass or staged during the weeks preceding the operation. In the latter procedure, preparation of erythrocyte concentrate, fresh frozen plasma, and even platelet rich plasma is possible. However, this involves a considerable investment in identification, storage, and general organisation (the patient has to be operated at the scheduled date, otherwise blood components may become outdated) is necessary. Furthermore, patients with coronary artery disease and angina pectoris are probably not the best candidates for major preoperative reduction of hematocrit. Medicamentous reactivation of platelets with desmopressin (Minirin) for improved hemostasis after cardiopulmonary bypass has been shown to have some effect. More convincing data has been published for the hemostatic effect of Aprotinin (Trasylol) in repeat open heart surgery by Royston et al (1987) and others.

A new approach is being evaluated at our institution in patients with normal or only slightly impaired left ventricular ejection fraction: platelet rich-plasma (800 ml) is withdrawn from the patient with a special spinning machine (Haemonetics PRP) during internal mammary artery take-down. The red cells are intermittently retransfused and the withdrawn volume is replaced continuously with saline. A cell saver is used during the coronary artery bypass procedure for maximum recovery of red cells. The concentrated red cells are retransfused whenever necessary whereas the platelet-rich plasma is retransfused after completed neutralization of heparin for improved hemostasis. Preliminary results are promising.

7.3.6.3 Improved Cardiopulmonary Bypass Equipment

Cardiopulmonary bypass equipment has been gradually improved over the last few years. The spinning disk oxygenator was abandoned a long time ago and has been replaced worldwide by disposable bubble oxygenators. The latter are now being replaced by integrated membrane oxygenators of modern design that allow independent adjustment of gas flow, FIO_2 and CO_2. Improved results of these devices, used either as closed or as open systems, in comparison to the classic bubble oxygenators have been demonstrated for cardiopulmonary bypass procedures of more than 2 h duration (von Segesser et al. 1987, 1990a). However there remain deleterious effects of prolonged cardiopulmonary bypass due to the moderate biocompatibility of the materials used. The necessity of systemic anticoagulation during cardiopulmonary bypass is one major contributing factor. Current developments include heparin-coated and heparin-like biomaterials. Canine studies on cardiopulmonary bypass with heparin surface-coated oxygenators and tubing sets performed at our institution without any systemic anticoagulation have shown reduced blood trauma and improved hemostasis (von Segesser and Turina 1989). The clinical studies in progress now at Zürich University Hospital have shown similar preliminary results (von Segesser et al. 1990).

7.3.7 Drainage

Because of the increased bleeding (Cosgrove et al. 1988) despite thorough hemostasis in bilateral internal mammary artery grafting adequate drainage of the pericardial sac and both pleural cavities is of prime importance. For this purpose an angulated chest tube (24 Fr) is placed behind the heart in the pericardial sac and another chest tube is placed at the deepest place of each pleural cavity. Occasionally, when the pleura can be maintained closed during internal mammary artery take-down or in cases with difficult hemostasis, a straight chest tube (28 Fr) is also placed in the anterior mediastinum. Before and after chest closure, but still in the sterile field, patency of all chest tubes is systematically checked with warm saline.

7.3.8 Closure of the Pericardial Sac and the Chest

Pericardial sac closure is not performed by all surgeons. However, complete closure of the pericardial sac after open-heart surgery has been reported to lower the incidence of complications at reoperation. In cases with complex internal mammary artery grafting this may not be realized systematically, but in most cases a plane of tissue can be interposed between the posterior surface of the sternum and the anterior surface of the heart and the great vessels, by adapting the two pleuropericardial flaps. Exceptionally, glutaraldehyde-preserved pericardial xenografts have been used for pericardial sac closure if no autologous tissue was available, e.g., in reoperations, after implant of synthetic grafts for reconstruction of the great vessels, or after resection of autologous pericardium for suture reinforcement (von Segesser et al. 1986b, 1987a). However, epicardial thickening, obscuring the coronary artery anatomy, as a reaction to the xenograft, has been reported and must be balanced before xenograft implantation.

The sternal borders are adapted with four separate figure-of-eight sutures made either from stainless steel wire, polyester suture material (Ethibond 5), or resorbable suture material (Maxon 5) and chest closure is completed in the usual fashion with a continuous running suture for the presternal fascia and a continuous running suture (resorbable or not) for the skin.

8 Results of Internal Mammary Artery–Coronary Artery Bypass Grafting

8.1 Early Results

8.1.1 Actual Series of Internal Mammary Artery–Coronary Artery Grafting

The internal mammary artery has been established as the preferred conduit for myocardial revascularization and the anatomical, pathological, and experimental data supporting its use as well as the indications, contraindications, and surgical techniques for take-down and construction of complex internal mammary artery–coronary artery revascularizations are discussed in the previous sections. This study was undertaken to analyze the actual results of clinical application of these concepts.

8.1.1.1 Material and Methods

A series of 114 consecutive patients operated upon by the same surgeon (L. v. S.) for coronary artery revascularization from March 1987 through March 1988 was analyzed. No patients undergoing coronary artery revascularization were excluded. Therefore the studied series includes elective coronary artery grafting, emergency coronary artery grafting, redo coronary artery grafting, and coronary artery grafting combined with valve surgery, resection of left ventricular aneurysm, aortic aneurysm, carotid endarterectomy and other procedures.

Both left and right internal mammary arteries were used for coronary artery revascularization when available and indicated. The revascularization was completed by saphenous vein grafts if necessary. Standard criteria and routine technique as described in Sect. 7. were applied throughout the study. Postoperative management included antiplatelet therapy (aspirin) for one year.

A total of 80 parameters summerizing patient variables as age, gender, medical history, surgical cardiovascular history, functional status, left ventricular function, extent of coronary artery disease, completeness of revascularization, outcome of surgery, including complications and postoperative follow-up were studied. The data were computerized, analyzed with the statistical package for social sciences as previously reported (von Segesser et al. 1986a) and cross tabulated. Quantitative data is given as mean ± standard deviation. Chi-square and Fisher's exact tests were used for categorical variables and Student's **t**-test was used to compare mean values when appropriate.

8.1.1.2 Results

8.1.1.2.1 Preoperative Variables

The analyzed series included 114 patients with a mean age of 56.5 ± 7.9 years (Fig. 85). 108 patients were male (94.7%) and 6 patients were female (5.3%). The medical history included the following risk factors and diagnoses at time of surgery: use of tobacco in 48 patients (42.1%), overweight (defined as body weight in kg more than 15% greater than height in cm −100) in 43 patients (37.7%), arterial hypertensive disease in 18 patients (15.8%), hyperlipemia in 13 patients (11.4%), insulin dependent diabetes in 2 patients (1.8%), and/or other diagnoses (including peripheral arterial disease, terminal renal failure, etc.) in 14 patients (12.3%) (Fig. 86). The surgical history included previous coronary artery revascularization in 2 patients with a mean interval of 8.5 ± 2.1 years between first and second operation. At first revascularization, both patient showed three-vessel disease and received 3 and 4 saphenous vein grafts.

At hospitalisation for the actual revascularization mean New York Heart Association functional status was assessed class I in 2 patients (1.8%), class II in 36 patients

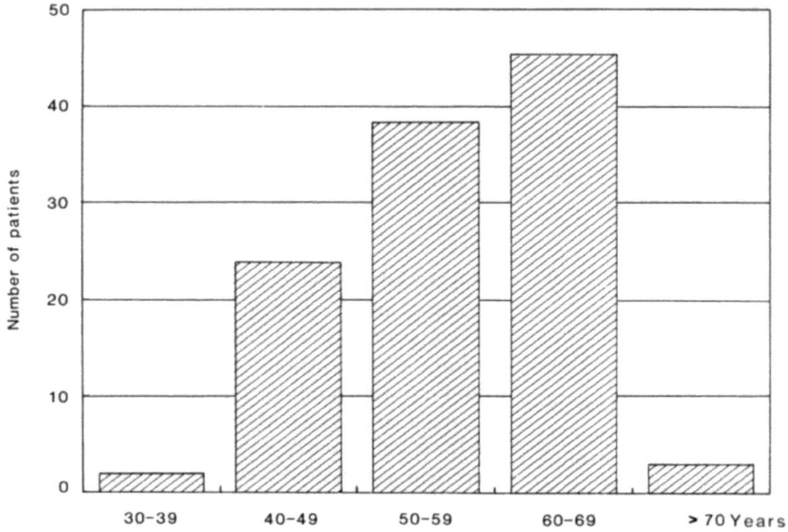

Fig. 85. Age at time of surgery (**n** = 114); mean age 56.5 ± 7.9 years)

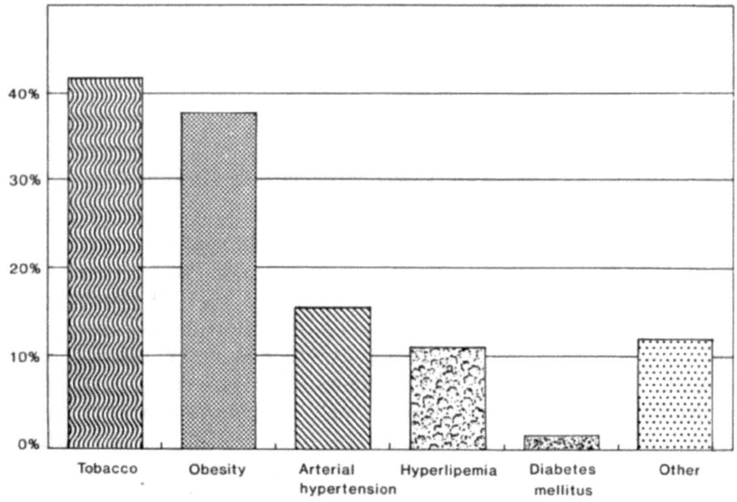

Fig. 86. Preoperative risk factors

(31.6%), class III in 63 patients (55.3%), and class IV in 13 patients (11.4%) (Fig. 87) or mean 2.8 ± 0.7. A total of 52 patients (45.6%) had suffered one previous infarction and 9 patients (7.9%) had suffered several previous infarctions. The interval between last myocardial infarction and surgery was less than 3 months in 10 patients: 8 weeks in 1 patient (0.9%), 3 weeks in 2 patients (1.8%), 1 week in 1 patient (0.9%), and less than 1 week in 6 patients (5.3%) for the patients operated upon on a scheduled basis. A total of 17 patients (14.9%) had no angina prior to surgery, whereas 84 patients (73.7%) suffered angina at stress test and 13 patients (11.4%) suffered angina at rest. Coronary artery revascularization was performed in 104 patients (91.2%) on a scheduled basis whereas in 10 patients (8.8%) surgery was performed as an emergency procedure. Indications for emergency procedures were failed percutaneous transluminal angioplasty (4), unstable angina and/or acute evolving myocardial infarction (4), and low cardiac output in patients with associated valve disease (2). In

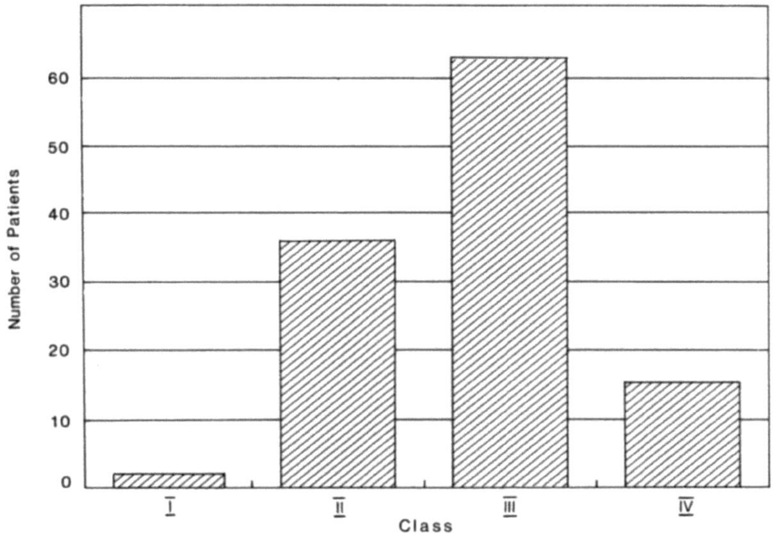

Fig. 87. Preoperative functional status according to the New York Heart Association classification

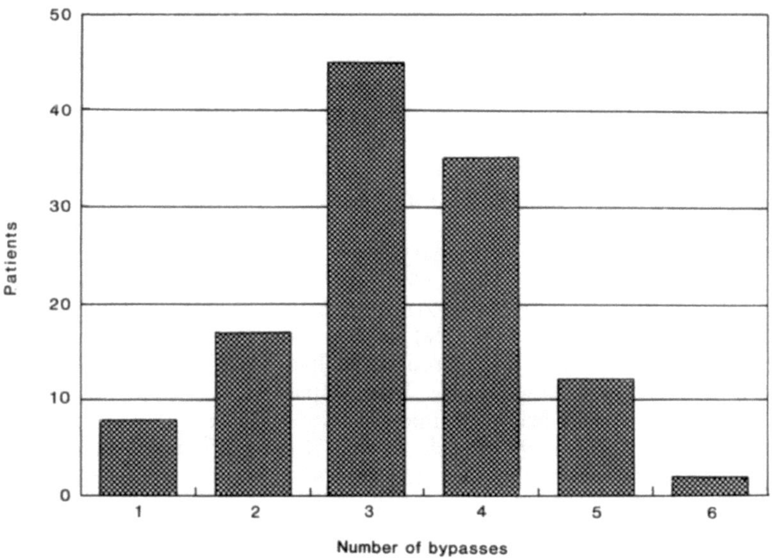

Fig. 88. Coronary artery revascularization; number of bypasses

the patients with scheduled operation preoperative stress test was positive (clinically and/or electrocardiographically) at a mean workload of 100±35 Watt. The coronary artery angiography revealed the following extent of coronary artery disease: single-vessel disease in 11 patients (9.6%), double-vessel disease in 19 patients (16.7%), and triple-vessel disease in 84 patients (73.7%). At time of catheterization, the left ventricular angiography showed mean ejection fraction of 55%±14% (range 25%–80%).

8.1.1.2.2 Operative Variables

A total number of 364 distal anastomoses for coronary artery revascularization was performed in the 114 operated patients; a mean bypass number of 3.2±1.1 per patient (range 1–6). Figure 88 shows the distribu-

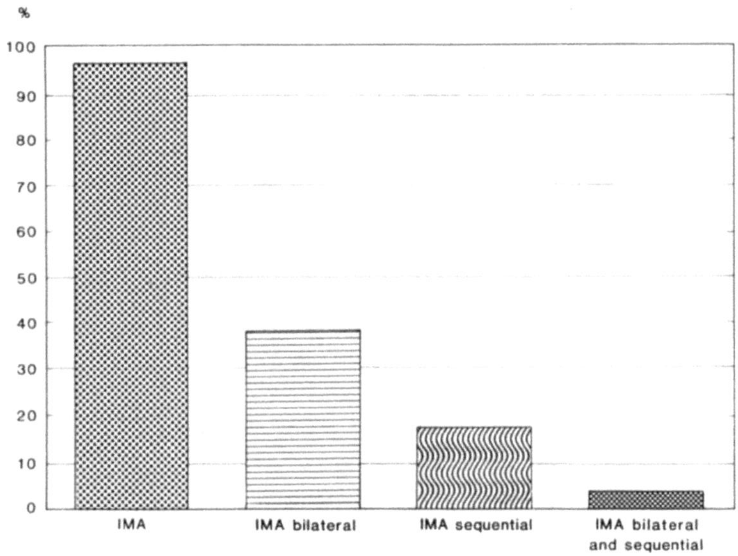

Fig. 89. Coronary artery revascularization; type of graft

tion as a function of the number of distal anastomoses: single bypass in 8 patients (7.0%), double bypass in 17 patients (14.9%), triple bypass in 45 patients (39.5%), quadruple bypass in 35 patients (30.7%), quintuple bypass in 12 patients (10.5%), and sextuple bypass in 2 patients (1.8%).

At least one internal mammary artery was used in 107/114 patients (93.9%); 101/104 scheduled operations (97.1%) and 6/10 emergency procedures (60.0%). In the 104 patients with scheduled operation, 96 had double- or triple-vessel disease. These 96 patients received at least one internal mammary artery graft in 93 procedures (96.9%), bilateral internal mammary artery grafts in 37 procedures (38.5%), sequential internal mammary artery grafts in 17 procedures (17.7%), and bilateral and sequential internal mammary artery grafts in 4 procedures (4.2%). Thus multiple internal mammary artery coronary artery grafting was performed in 50/96 patients or 52.0% (Fig. 89).

Major contraindications for internal mammary artery grafting in the complete series included either isolated or combined: emergency procedure (5), coagulopathy (4), low left ventricular ejection fraction (3), and internal mammary artery stenosis (1). Associated procedures such as valve replacement (6), resection of left ventricular aneurysm (3), resection of infrarenal aortic aneurysm (1) and endarteriectomy of carotid bifurcation (1) were not considered to be contraindications for internal mammary artery grafting.

Distribution of grafts throughout the complete series was as follows. Revascularization of the left anterior descending coronary artery was performed in 112 cases (98.2%): with an internal mammary artery in 105 procedures (92%) and with a saphenous vein graft in 7 procedures (6.1%). Revascularization of a diagonal branch was performed in 50 cases (43.9%): with an internal mammary artery graft in 15 procedures (13.2%) and with a saphenous vein graft in 35 procedures (30.7%). Revascularization of the left circumflex coronary artery was performed in 83 cases (72.8%): with an internal mammary artery in 2 procedures (1.8%) and with a saphenous vein graft in 81 procedures (71.1%). The obtuse marginal branch was revascularized in 32 cases (28%) with a saphenous vein graft. The right coronary artery was revascularized in 70 cases (61.4%): with an internal mammary artery graft in 31 procedures (27.2%) and with a saphenous vein graft in 49 procedures (43.0%). The right posterior descending coronary artery was revascularized in 7 cases (6.1%): with an internal mammary artery graft in 4 procedures (3.5%) and with a saphenous vein graft in 3 procedures (2.6%). Revascularization of marginal branches originating from the right coronary artery system was tabulated with the circumflex coronary artery system as they were in general revascularized by the same sequential saphenous vein graft.

The relative proportion of internal mammary artery grafts in relation to all grafts used for revascularization of a coronary artery is depicted in Fig. 90.

The quality of the available vein grafts was assessed in 74 patients as good (64.9%) and in 40 patients as mediocre (35.1%).

Endarterectomy of the right coronary artery system was performed in 3 cases (2.4%).

8.1.1.2.3 Postoperative Variables

8.1.1.2.3.1 Mortality

There were 2 hospital deaths in the entire series. Hospital mortality for elective coronary artery revascularization was 1/104 (0.96%) whereas it was 1/10 (10%) for the emergency revascularization procedures (Fig. 91).

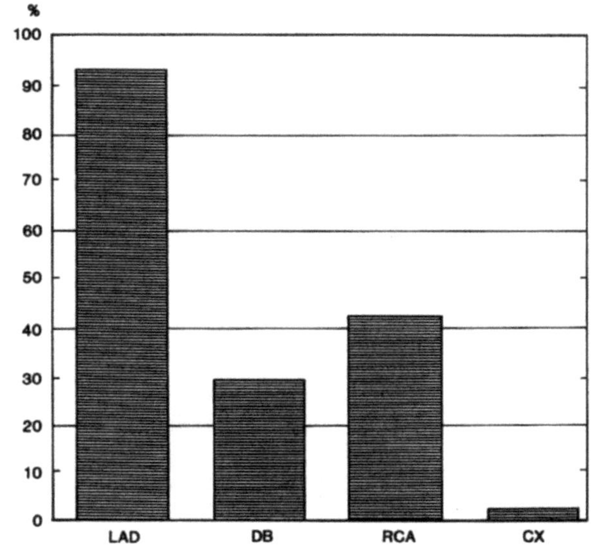

Fig. 90. Proportion of internal mammary artery grafts used for revascularization of the different coronary arteries as a percentage of the anastomoses performed (LAD: left anterior descending coronary artery; DB: diagonal branch; RCA: right coronary artery; CX: left circumflex coronary artery)

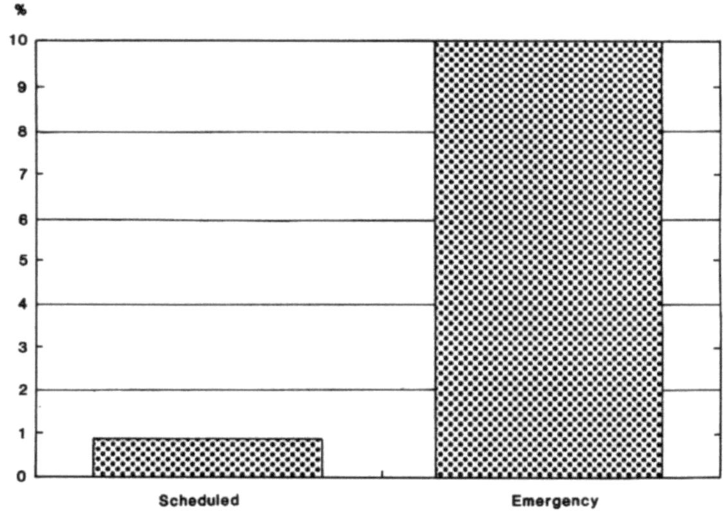

Fig. 91. Mortality for scheduled and emergency procedures

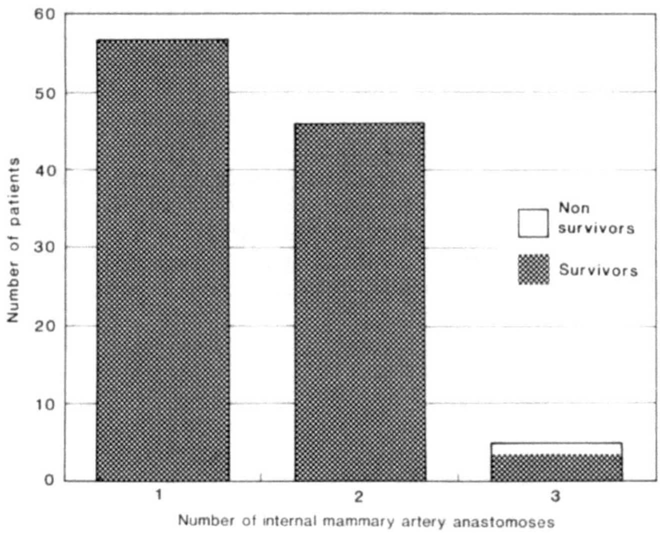

Fig. 92. Mortality as a function of the number of internal mammary artery anastomoses

As a function of the used grafts, hospital mortality was 1/107 (0.93%) for patients revascularized with at least one internal mammary artery graft in comparison to 1/7 (14.2%) for patients revascularized with saphenous vein grafts only (because of contraindications for revascularization with internal mammary artery grafts such as failed percutaneous transluminal angioplasty).

As a function of the number of constructed internal mammary artery–coronary artery anastomoses constructed, hospital mortality was 0/57 cases with 1 internal mammary artery–coronary artery anastomosis, 0/46 cases with two internal mammary artery–coronary artery anastomoses and 1/4 cases with three internal mammary artery–coronary artery anastomoses (Fig. 92).

Figure 93 shows the postmortem angiography with six patent anastomoses, of the only death in the series of elective procedures. Significant left ventricular hypertrophia (Fig. 94) and severe myocardial sclerosis of the left ventricular wall must have contributed to the pump failure in this case. The second nonsurvivor belongs to the series of emergency procedures due to failed percutaneous transluminal angioplasty. The patient had a cardiac arrest in the catheterization lab and was brought to the operating theater under external massage. Despite immediate connection to the pump oxygenator by femorofemoral cannulation and construction of three saphenous vein grafts to the main coronary arteries he could never be weaned from cardiopulmonary bypass. Postmortem angiogram showed 3 patent grafts.

8.1.1.2.3.2 Morbidity

The morbidity of the survivors is depicted in Fig. 95. Bleeding complications leading to reoperation were recorded in seven patients (6.1%). Ten revisions of the operating field were performed: six times in three patients for excessive bleeding, three times in three patients for established tamponade and once in one patient for exclusion of tamponade. In one patient tamponade occurred on the third postoperative day after mobilization. At rethoracotomy, the right internal mammary artery graft was found to be interrupted at about 1 cm above the distal anastomosis onto the right posterior descending coronary artery, but the distal anastomosis was intact. This in situ internal mammary artery pedicle was obviously too short for the descended heart in the upright position. Emergency rethoracotomy allowed successful control of bleeding, but led to a prolonged hospital stay because of sternal wound healing problems.

Major wound complications leading to

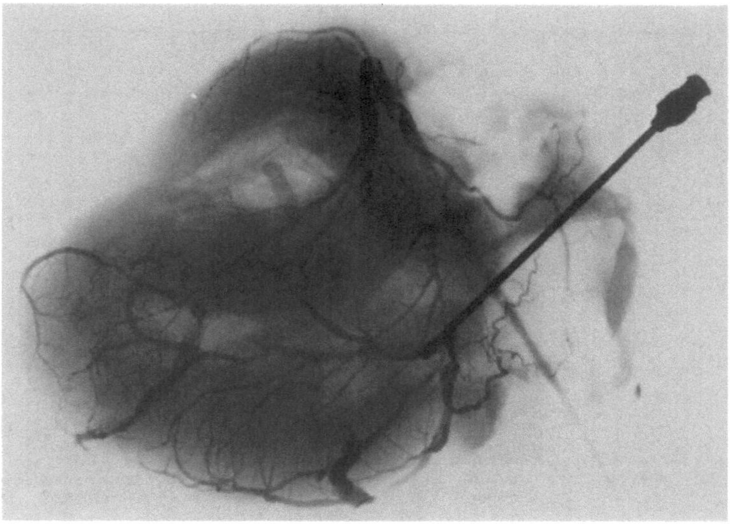

Fig. 93. Postmortem angiography showing six patent coronary artery bypass grafts

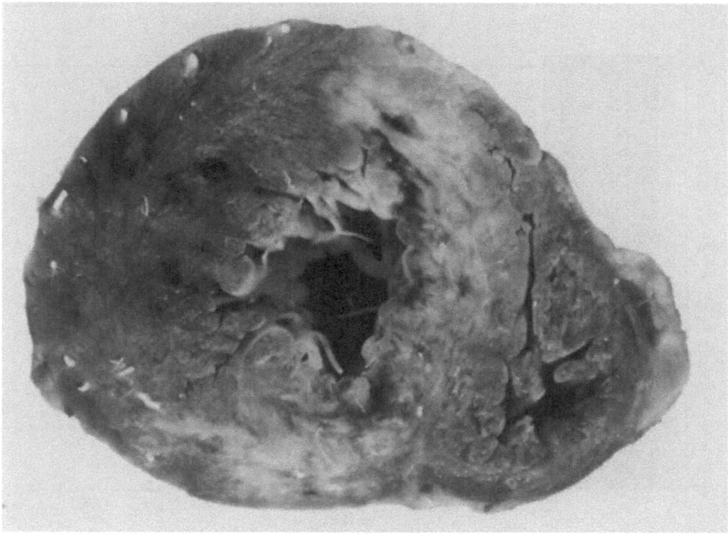

Fig. 94. Transverse section of the heart showing significant left ventricular hypertrophia (same case as Fig. 93)

surgical debridement, sternal refixation, and implantation of gentamicin beads (von Segesser et al. 1988) were observed in 3/114 patients (2.6%). In one diabetic patient secondary healing could only be achieved by the means of plastic surgery (rotation of musculus pectoralis major).

Mechanical circulatory support by means of the intra-aortic balloon pump was necessary in one surviving patient (1/110: 0.9%).

Peroperative infarctions were diagnosed in 3/112 survivors (2.7%) by two or more of the following criteria: creatine kinase more than three times normal and myocardial fraction (CK-MB) more than 10%, significant Q-wave in ECG and impaired ventricular function in postoperative bidimensional echocardiography, angiogram, or isotope study. Postoperative coronary artery catheterization showed occlusion of a saphenous vein graft in two patients and no flow in an internal mammary artery graft in one patient. Infarction in relation to the type of graft occurred in 2/37 patients with bilat-

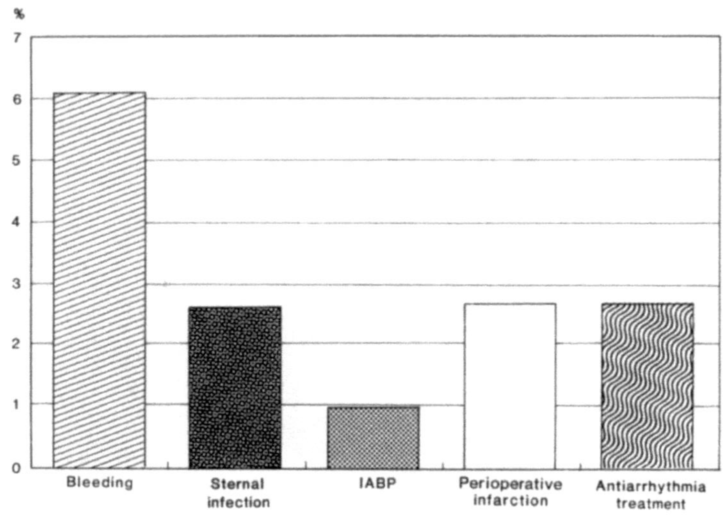

Fig. 95. Morbidity of coronary artery revascularization with systematical use of internal mammary artery grafts

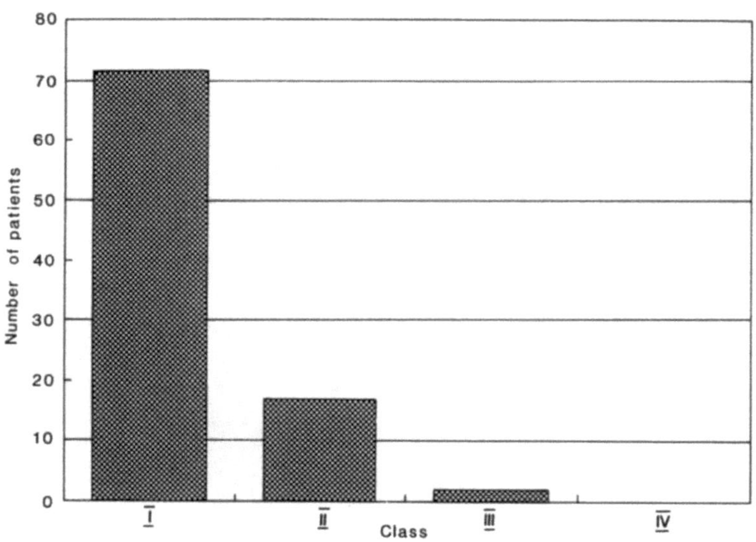

Fig. 96. Postoperative functional status according to the New York Heart Association classification.

eral internal mammary artery grafts and in 1/17 patients with sequential internal mammary artery graft. Antiarrhythmic treatment at hospital discharge was necessary in three patients (2.7%). Mean hospital stay for the entire series was 7.9±4.0 days.

8.1.1.2.3.3 Follow-up

After a mean follow-up of 5.5±3.7 months a total of 93/110 survivors could be controlled (85%). At that time New York Heart Association functional status was assessed (mean 1.23±0.47). A total of 72 patients (79.1%) were in class I, 17 patients (18.7%) were in class II and 2 patients (1.8%) were in class III as shown in Fig. 96. After the operation, 80% of the patients were free from angina. There is a significant diffrence between mean preoperative New York Heart Association functional class of 2.76±0.67 and mean postoperative functional class of 1.23±0.47 (**P** < 0.0005).

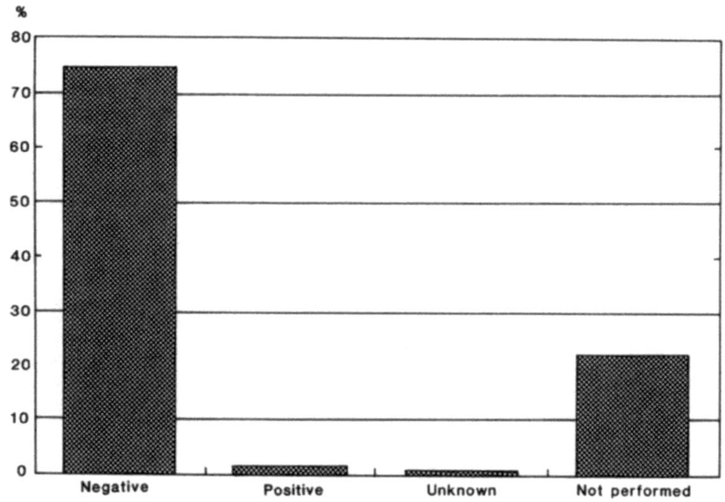

Fig. 97. Stress test after myocardial revascularization with at least one internal mammary artery–coronary artery anastomosis in 94% of operated cases

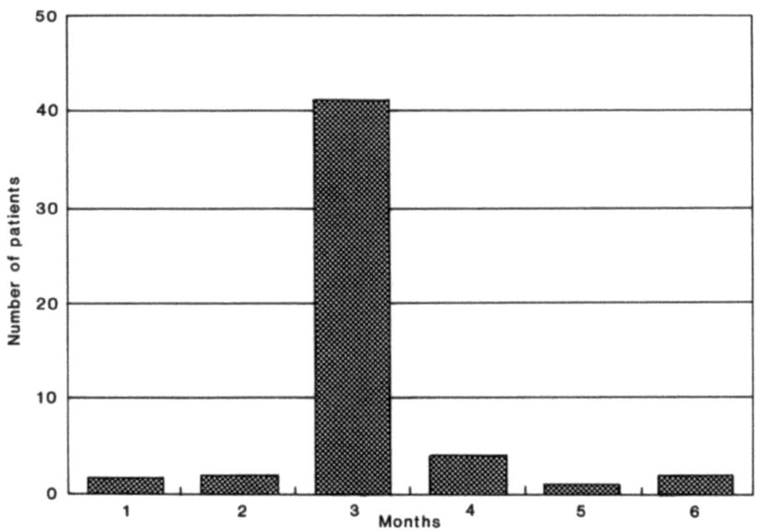

Fig. 98. Return to work after coronary artery revascularization of 79 analyzed patients: mean interval 2.9±1.0 months

Stress test (cycloergometer) was negative in 84 survivors (75.0%), positive (clinically and electrocardiographically) in 2 (1.8%), of unknown result in 1 (0.9%), and missing in 25 (22.3%) as depicted in Fig. 97. Mean achieved workload was 122±32 W. This has to be compared to the preoperative stress test which was positive in all patients at a mean work-load of 100±35 W (**P**<0.0005).

After a mean interval of 2.9±1.0 months 53/79 analyzed patients (67%) had resumed work. The interval between operation and return to work is depicted in Fig. 98. There were 65 operated patients less than 60 years of age. In this group return to work could be assessed in 50/65 (77%). Of fifty patients, 38 (76%) had resumed work at time of follow-up whereas 11/50 (22%) had not and 1/50 (2%) was retired (Fig. 99).

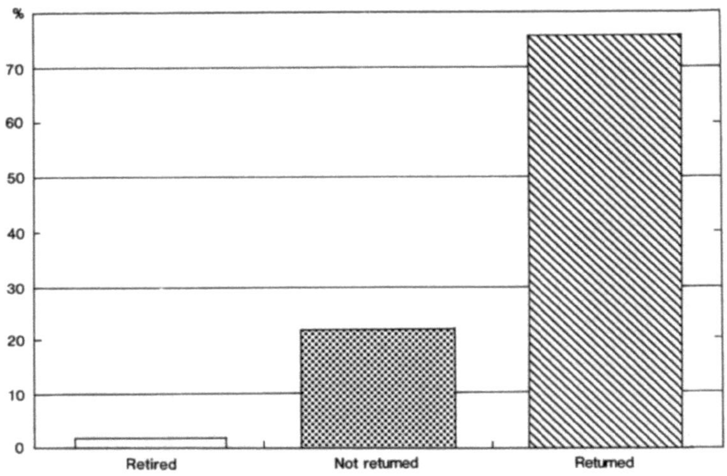

Fig. 99. Return to work of patients less than 60 years of age

8.1.2 Early Results of Expanded Internal Mammary Artery Grafting in Comparison to Classic Saphenous Vein Grafting

Early results of internal mammary artery grafting in comparison to classic saphenous vein grafting were previously analyzed by von Segesser et al. (1986a). In a series of 100 consecutive patients the internal mammary arteries were used for coronary artery revascularization whenever indicated. At least one internal mammary artery was used in 89% of cases; both internal mammary arteries were used in 30%, and in 17% sequential internal mammary artery–coronary artery anastomoses were constructed. The results in this group of patients were compared to another group of 250 consecutive patients in whom the coronary arteries were revascularized by classic saphenous vein grafts. In-hospital mortality was 3% for the internal mammary artery group and 2.5% for the saphenous vein group (no significant difference). The follow-up was complete for 89% of the patients after a mean duration of 6 months. At follow-up, the New York Heart Association mean functional class was assessed 1.0 ± 0.2 for the internal mammary artery group and 1.2 ± 0.2 for the saphenous vein group ($\mathbf{P} < 0.01$). Stress test was electrocardiographically positive in 7.1% of the internal mammary artery group and in 15.3% of the saphenous vein group ($\mathbf{P} < 0.05$). Although internal mammary artery grafting is more demanding in comparison to saphenous vein grafting, the early results appeared to be superior for the former in comparison to the latter.

The risk of bilateral internal mammary artery grafting was analyzed by Cosgrove et al. (1988) in three groups of patients who were computer-matched for recognized risk factors: year of operation, age, gender, extent of coronary artery disease, left ventricular function, completeness of myocardial revascularization, and history of congestive heart failure as reported in Sect. 6.2.3. The patient groups differed in the fact that they received veins only, one internal mammary artery graft, or two internal mammary artery grafts. The operative mortality rates for these three groups were 1.8%, 0.3%, and 0.9% respectively (no significant difference). Analysis of perioperative morbidity demonstrated no significant differences except an increase in transfusion requirements in the group receiving two internal mammary artery grafts ($\mathbf{P} = 0.04$).

As previously pointed out, this study is not randomized and the authors do not report why some patients received only vein grafts while others received internal mammary artery grafts. The trend is to place vein grafts in a group of patients with less favorable, unmatched, preoperative variables. In this study, the final similar outcome for all groups shows that for such cases, with a sum of unfavorable variables, saphenous vein grafting should be preferred. However, one has to admit that the overall mortality and morbidity for the three matched groups are in the same range even if minor differences in less recognized risk factors are not matched.

8.1.3 Evolution of Perioperative Mortality in Coronary Artery Revascularization

Overall thirty-day mortality in 3397 patients undergoing coronary artery revascularization at Zürich University Hospital from 1978 through 1987 was analyzed by Lioupis (1988). The series consisted of 3075 men (90.5%) and 322 women (9.5%). The women were significantly older than the men (mean age 56.5±9.1 versus 54.4±7.2 years: **P** < 0.001). The mean age increased from 52.8 years for women and 52.2 years for men in 1978 to 60.6 and 57.0 years respectively in 1987. Typical angina was present in 2653 patients (78.0%), whereas unstable angina was noted in 601 patients (17.7%), and 143 patients (4.3%) had no chest pain. Previous myocardial infarctions were recorded in 1743 patients (51.3), 86 were reoperation cases (2.5%), and 299 (8.8%) underwent nonelective operations. Most of the patients (90.0%) had two- (17.7%) or three-vessel disease (72.3%) and preoperative ejection fraction of 50% or more was recorded in 86.5%. The number of patients with quadruple or more bypass grafts increased from 6.8% in 1978 to 45% in 1987. The proportion of internal mammary artery bypass grafting increased from 1/146 (0.7%) in 1978 to 87/472 (18.4%) unilateral internal mammary artery bypass grafts and 2/472 (0.4%) bilateral internal mammary artery bypass grafts in 1984 to reach 270/378 (71.4%) unilateral internal mammary artery grafts and 76/378 (20.1%) bilateral internal mammary artery grafts in 1987 as depicted in Fig. 100.

Overall 30–day mortality was 1% (confidence limits: 0.8%–1.2%); 30–day mortality increased significantly with decreased ejection fraction: 1.6% with ejection fraction between 30% and 49% and 11.1% with ejection fraction below 30% (**P** < 0.001). Significantly higher 30–day mortality was also associated with: left mainstem stenosis (3.8%; **P** < 0.005), nonelective procedures (3.7%; **P** < 0.001) and redoprocedures (5.8%; **P** < 0.001). The following factors increased the probability of perioperative mortality without reaching statistical significance: age > 70 years (2%; **P** > 0.25), female gender (1.9%; **P** > 0.05), number of grafted vessels (0.6–1.4%; **P** > 0.25), aortic cross clamp time (**P** > 0.25), severity of angina (New York Heart Association functional class I and II: 0.7%; **P** > 0.1; class IV: 1.7%: **P** > 0.05) and previous myocardial infarction (1.2%: **P** > 0.1). The most common cause of death was myocardial in-

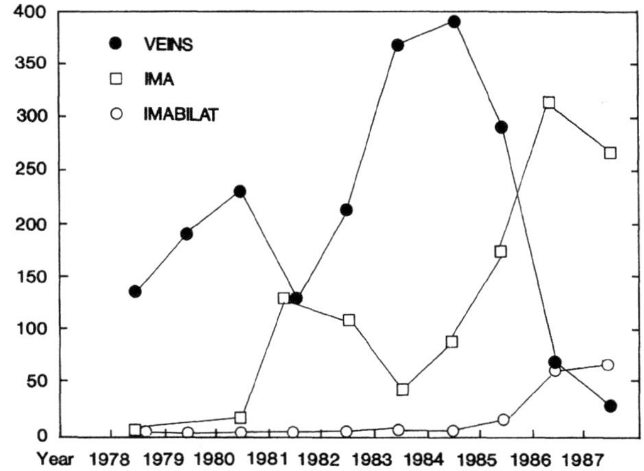

Fig. 100. Proportion of internal mammary artery grafting over 10 years of coronary artery revascularization

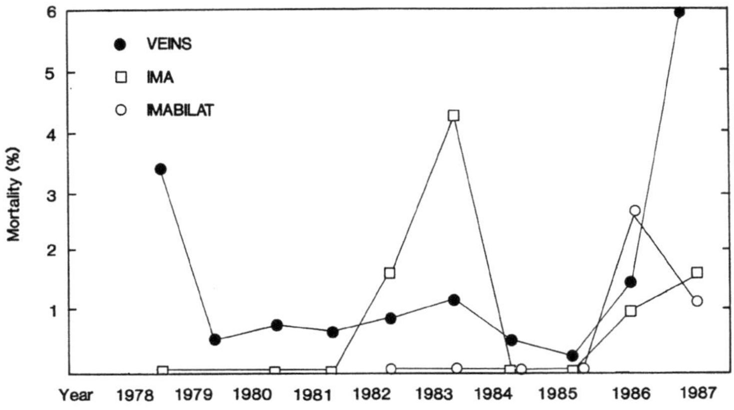

Fig. 101. Overall 30-day mortality in function of selected graft: after 1985, mortality increases in the group revascularized with saphenous vein grafts only, because of more high-risk patients in this group.

farction in 19/34 deaths (55.9%). Figure 101 shows 30–day mortality as a function of selected graft. For patients revascularized with saphenous vein grafts 30-day mortality was 21/2053 patients (1.0%) compared to 11/1174 patients (0.94%) for patients revascularized with one internal mammary artery and 2/170 patients (1.2%) for patients revascularized with both internal mammary arteries. There is no statistically significant difference in respect of 30-day mortality, whether none, one or both internal mammary arteries are used for revascularization in these series.

8.2 Medium-Term Results of Internal Mammary Artery–Coronary Artery Grafting

Medium-term results of expanded internal mammary artery grafting in comparison to multivessel coronary artery angioplasty were analyzed by Finci et al. (1987b).

8.2.1 Patients and Methods

The study comprised 80 consecutive patients who underwent surgical myocardial revascularization with both internal mammary arteries, and 80 patients who underwent multivessel percutaneous transluminal coronary angioplasty. In the surgical group, additional vein grafts were used whenever necessary for completion of revascularization. Preoperative patients characteristics for the two groups are given in Fig. 102.

Surgical revascularization of the coronary arteries was performed by means of both internal mammary arteries in all patients. The internal mammary arteries were used as pedicled conduits in all cases and the anastomoses were constructed as priviously reported (von Segesser et al. 1986a). The type of anastomoses performed with the left and right internal mammary arteries are shown in Fig. 103.

Multivessel percutaneous transluminal coronary angioplasty was defined as angioplasty during one session of at least two of the following vessels: left anterior descending coronary artery, left circumflex coronary artery, right coronary artery, or coronary artery bypass graft. The distribution of the vessels dilated during one session is given in Fig. 103.

Clinical follow-up consisted of an interview and/or exercise stress test. It was available in all patients at a mean interval of 16±9 months after surgery and 12±6 months for patients with angioplasty. Exercise tests were carried out according to a bicycle exercise protocol with a Marquette Electronics Inc. computer assisted system. Tests were started at a workload of 25 W

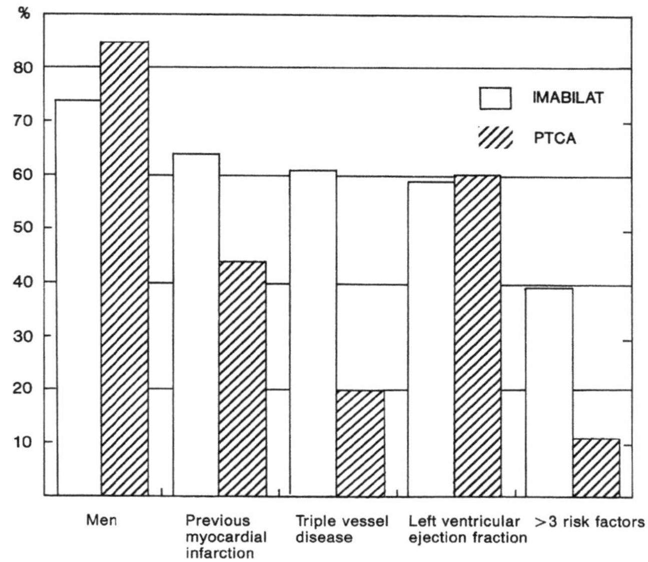

Fig. 102. Patient characteristics

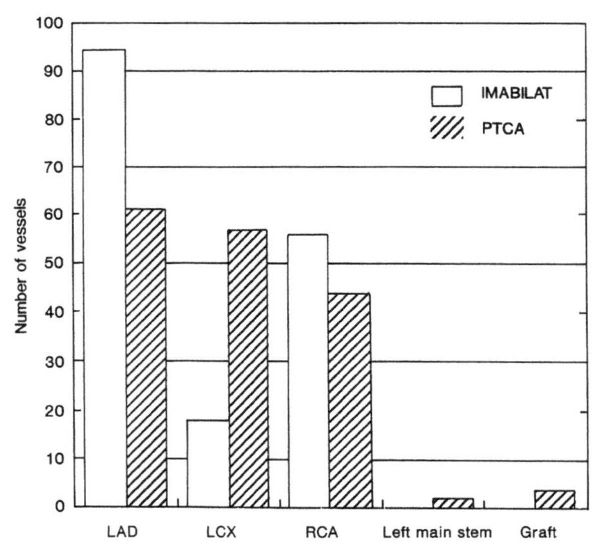

Fig. 103. Revascularized vessels (LAD: left anterior descending coronary artery; LCX: left circumflex coronary artery; RCA: right coronary artery)

with increments of 25 W every 3 minutes up to the maximal calculated workload or target heart rate, unless significant ST segment depression (> 0.1 mV) or chest pain appeared. The time from the start of exercise until 0.1 mV ST segment depression (0.08 ms from the J-point) was recorded. Two main functional variables of the exercise test performance were evaluated in all patients: maximal workload (in W) and double product (maximal blood pressure × maximal heart rate, in mmHg × beats/min/100). Antianginal drugs were not withheld. All values are expressed as mean ± standard deviation. Differences were analyzed with Student's **t**-test for paired or unpaired variables, respectively, or the chi-square test where appropriate. A **P** value of less than 0.05 was considered significant.

8.2.2 Results

In patients with surgery 2.7 distal anastomoses per patient were performed, and in patients with percutaneous transluminal coronary angioplasty a mean of 2.2 vessels per patient were attempted. Primary success of percutaneous transluminal coronary angioplasty was 86% versus 94% for surgery. Overall complicationrate was 7% for patients in the angioplasty group versus 6% for patients in the surgical group. Control angiograms, done in 86% of patients (59/69) after successful angioplasty, showed a recurrence in 42% (15/59). Repeat percutaneous transluminal angioplasty was done in 15, elective surgery in 7, and a medical treatment was pursued in 3 patients with

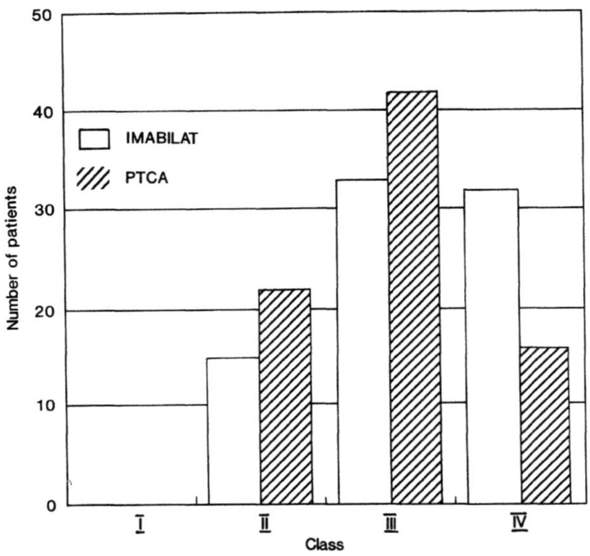

A

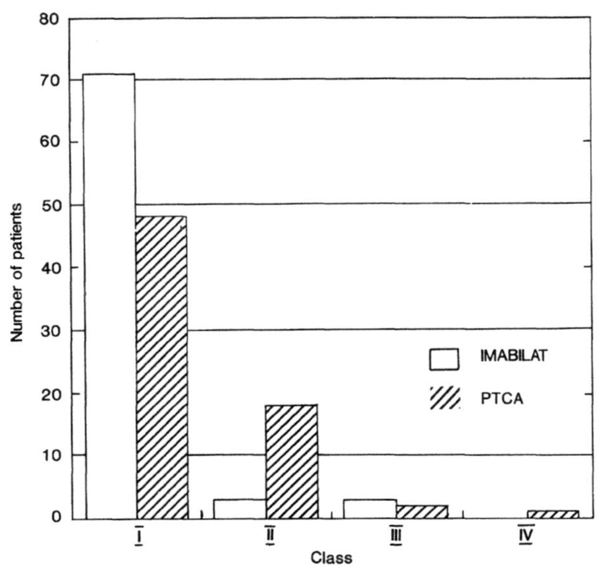

B

Fig. 104. New York Heart Association functional status before (**A**) and after (**B**) coronary artery revascularization

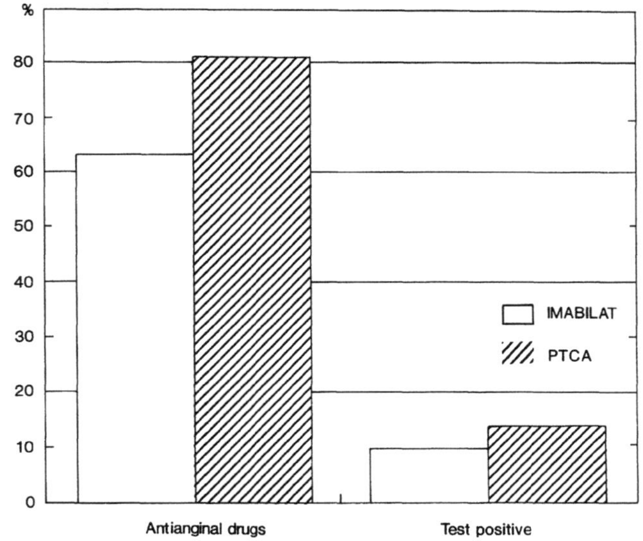

Fig. 105. Exercise test performance after revascularization; results at follow-up after 1 year or more

restenosis. Recurrence of symptoms after successful surgery was found in 3 patients (4%). They were treated with percutaneous transluminal angioplasty. Mean improvement of New York Heart Association functional status was 2.1 classes after surgery and 1.5 classes after successful angioplasty (Fig. 104); 89% (71/80) versus 60% (48/80), were in class I (**P** < 0.0001). There were more surgical patients than angioplasty patients without antianginal drugs at follow-up: 37% (18/38) versus 19% (11/58); **P** < 0.05, and their double product during exercise testing was superior (295 ± 57 versus 272 ± 56 mmHg × beats/min/100; **P** < 0.05) as shown in Fig. 105.

8.2.3 Comments

Unequal baseline variables are an important limitation of this nonrandomized study. There was a higher extent of coronary artery disease (Fig. 102) in surgical patients compared with patients who underwent angioplasty (triple vessel disease in 61% and 20%, respectively), as well as a higher prevalence of previous myocardial infarction (64% and 44%, respectively) and three or more risk factors (39% and 11% respectively). Furthermore, most of the patients were recommended for surgery only after having been considered for angioplasty and rejected. Primary success and complication rates including mortality were similar in both groups. There is a lack of angiographic documentation of patency of the bypass grafts in the surgical group. Thus, some additional surgical failures may have gone unrecognized. Nonetheless, the finding that there was a higher symptomatic improvement in the surgical group appears clear. The medium-term results were favorable for both techniques of multivessel revascularization. The mean functional improvement after successful surgical revascularization was 2.1 New York Heart Association classes. This is better than the improvement of 1.5 classes after successful angioplasty (Fig. 104). This may be explained by the more compromised initial functional status of the surgical patients. However, the fact that 89% versus 60% of patients were in New York Heart Association functional class I at follow-up is clearly in favor of bypass surgery.

Improvement of exercise performance reached high significance in both groups. However, 42% of patients after a first angioplasty had an angiographic recurrence of at least one lesion. With primary success of 86% and documented restenosis of 31% (25/80) only 55% (44/80) of patients had a possible sustained benefit after the initial angioplasty, when further invasive procedures are disregarded, while this figure amounts to 89% (71/80) in the surgical group.

Percutaneous transluminal coronary angioplasty on the other hand seems to offer an advantage in terms of cost and morbidity even considering patients with repeat angioplasty after recurrence of stenosis. Repeat angioplasty has therefore to be included as an integral part of percutaneous transluminal coronary angioplasty to render its medium-term results comparable to those of bypass surgery. Yet the functional outcome of the surgical patients revascularized with both internal mammary arteries is still superior.

Similar results were found by Hochberg et al. (1989) in a retrospective study comparing matched series with coronary angioplasty versus coronary bypass over three years. Patient evaluation revealed that 63% (76/121) of the angioplasty group were alive and in New York Heart Association class I or II 3 years after one or two angioplasty procedures. This figure compares with 92% (110/120) of surgical patients alive and in the same two New York Heart Association classes (**P** < 0.0000).

Percutaneous transluminal coronary angioplasty ($n = 389$) and coronary artery bypass grafting ($n = 1000$) as initial nonemergency treatment strategies were analyzed retrospectively by Akins et al. (1989). Hospital mortality rates for coronary bypass grafting and angioplasty were 0.4% and 0.5%, respectively, and infarction rates were 1.7% and 5.1%, respectively (**P** < 0.01). Freedom from all morbidity and mortality at 5 years 87.1% for coronary bypass grafting versus 66.0% for angioplasty (**P** < 0.001). By Cox regression analysis for all 1389 patients, only diminished ejection fraction and advanced age predicted poor long-term survival (**P** < 0.001). The only significant predictor of nonfatal late events was having had coronary angioplasty.

8.3 Late Results of Internal Mammary Artery–Coronary Artery Grafting

Late survival after internal mammary artery grafting in comparison to venous grafting is shown in Table 4. The results reported in the literature were compiled to obtain a mean survival rate ± standard deviation as a function of the graft used. The survival rate after internal mammary artery grafting in general was 97.6% ± 1.9% at 30 days (13 studies), 95.3% ± 5.5% at 1 year (4 studies), 91.2% ± 3.1% at 5 years (6 studies), 86.6% ± 5.6% at 10 years (4 studies), and 72% at 14 years as compared to saphenous vein grafting with 97.1% ± 2.7% at 30 days (5 studies), 92.3% ± 5.5% at 1 year (3 studies), 89.2% ± 2.5% at 5 years (3 studies), 77.7% ± 9.6% at 10 years (3 studies), and 57% after 14 years (see Fig. 106).

Improved survival rates with internal mammary artery grafting in comparison to saphenous vein grafting were reported in all studies addressing the question and appear also after compiling the mean survival rates for the different types of grafts at the various intervals of follow-up. Mean follow-up rate for all tabulated studies was 97.8% ± 7.2% for 42 analyzed subsets of patients with complete data and was not available in 23 analyzed subsets.

The survival rate of expanded internal mammary artery grafting, defined as more than one internal mammary artery anastomosis (sequential internal mammary artery grafts, bilateral internal mammary artery grafts, and/or free internal mammary artery grafts) was as follows: 97.0% ± 4.0% at 30 days (13 studies), 94.2% ± 5.7% at 1 year (4 studies), 95.1% ± 6.9% at 5 years (2 studies), 81.1% ± 11.0% at 10 years (2 studies) and 86.0% at 14 years (Fig. 107). The apparent increase in survival rate with time is due to the different number of studies at the different intervals. The plotted mean survival rates are similar to those observed with unilateral internal mammary artery grafting and better than those reported with saphenous vein grafting (Fig. 108). However, the study for bilateral internal mammary artery grafting performed by Cameron et al. (1986) shows the best survival rates at 14 years in comparison to unilateral internal mammary

Table 4. Survival rate

Reference	Type of graft and vessel	Follow-up (mean)	No. of patients	Control rate (%)	Survival rate (%)
Collins et al. 1973	Veins	30 days	180	100	94.5
Loop et al. 1973	LIMA–LAD, LCX + veins	30 days	175	100	99.0
		10 months	100	57	99.0
Suzuki et al. 1973	IMA bilat + veins	30 days	43	100	95.3
Kay et al. 1974	IMA–LAD, LCX, RCA + veins	30 days	628	100	94.9
Barner 1974a	IMA bilat	30 days	100	100	92.0
Grondin et al. 1975	Veins	30 days	100	100	94.0
		1 year	100	100	92.0
	IMA	30 days	40	100	98.0
		1 year	40	100	97.0
Green et al. 1979	IMA	30 days	140	100	98.6
		5 years		100	93.0
Lytle et al. 1980	LIMA–LAD	30 days	100	100	100
		55 months	100	90	98
	Vein–LAD	30 days	100	100	100
		77 months	100	90	98
Tyras et al. 1980	LIMA–LAD	30 days	765	100	98.6
		5 years		?	87.6
	Vein–LAD	30 days	694	100	98.1
		5 years		?	88.7
Chassignolle et al. 1982	LIMA–LAD + Veins	30 days	350	100	96.0
		4 years	100	?	87.1
		6 years	350	?	87.8
Hanna et al. 1983	IMA + veins	30 days	1000	100	98.8
Tector et al. 1983	IMA + veins	30 days	298	100	99.3
		7 years	298	?	91.6
Harjola et al. 1984	IMA sequent + veins	30 days	61	100	96.6
Okies et al. 1984	IMA + veins	30 days	259	?	99.0
		5 years	295	?	92.0
		10 years	295	?	82.0
	Veins	30 days	139	?	99.0
		5 years	139	?	87.0
		10 years	139	?	69.0
Tector et al. 1984	IMA sequent + veins	30 days	29	100	100
		1 year	29	100	96.6
Cosgrove et al. 1985c	IMA + veins	5 years	x/1000	?	95.6
		10 years	x/1000	?	85.8
	Veins	5 years	1000 – x	?	92.0
		10 years	1000 – x	?	76.2
Kamath et al. 1985	IMA sequent unilat	21 months	49	100	97.9
	IMA bilat sequent unilat		31	100	96.7
	IMA sequent bilat		7	100	85.7

Table 4. (Continued)

Reference	Type of graft and vessel	Follow-up (mean)	No. of patients	Control rate (%)	Survival rate (%)
Cameron et al. 1986	IMA unilat + veins	5 years	494	97	91.2
		10 years	494	89	81.9
		14 years	494	?	72.0
	IMA bilat + veins	5 years	38	97	100
		10 years	38	89	88.9
		14 years	38	?	86.0
	Veins	14 years	216	?	57.0
Coll-Mazzei et al. 1986	Veins	30 days	126	100	98.3
		10 years	126	100	68.0
Loop et al. 1986a	LIMA-LAD + veins	10 years	2306	?	93.4
	Veins	10 years	3625	?	88.0
Loop et al. 1986b	Free IMA + veins	30 days	156	100	99.4
		5 years	156	?	90.2
		10 years	156	?	73.3
Lytle et al. 1986	IMA bilat + veins	30 days	500	100	98.6
Olearchyk and Magovern 1986	LIMA-LAD	30 days	833	100	97.8
		10 years	833	?	89.0
Rankin et al. 1986	Expanded IMA				
	scheduled	30 days	x/466	100	99.6
	emergency	30 days	466−x	100	96.9
von Segesser et al. 1986a	Expanded IMA + veins	30 days	100	100	97.0
	Veins	30 days	250	100	97.5
Tector et al. 1986	Expanded IMA + veins	30 days	100	100	99.0
von Segesser Sect. 8.1.1	Expanded IMA + veins	30 days	104	100	99.0

The tabulated figures were calculated from the data available in the studies cited. However, indications, surgical techniques, and data analyses may differ from one study to another.
IMA internal mammary artery; LIMA left internal mammary artery; RIMA right internal mammary artery; unilat unilateral; bilat bilateral; sequent sequential anastomoses; LAD left anterior descending coronary artery; LCX left circumflex coronary artery; RCA right coronary artery; ? actual percentage of controlled patients could not be assessed (in general actuarial analyses)

artery grafting and saphenous vein grafting (Fig. 109). On the other hand, the results of free internal mammary artery grafting at 10 years (survival rate 73.3%) are inferior to the compiled results of saphenous vein grafting (77.7%), inferior to the compiled results of internal mammmary artery grafting in general (86.6%), and inferior to the available results on bilateral internal mammary artery grafting (88.9%) which are the best (Fig. 110).

Based on the reported long-term (10 years and more) survival rates, the individual as well as the compiled figures, and our own data, the best available technique for coronary artery revascularization appears to be bilateral internal mammary artery grafting, followed by unilateral internal mammary artery grafting.

The value of the free internal mammary artery graft is still difficult to assess as the late results are worse than one would expect

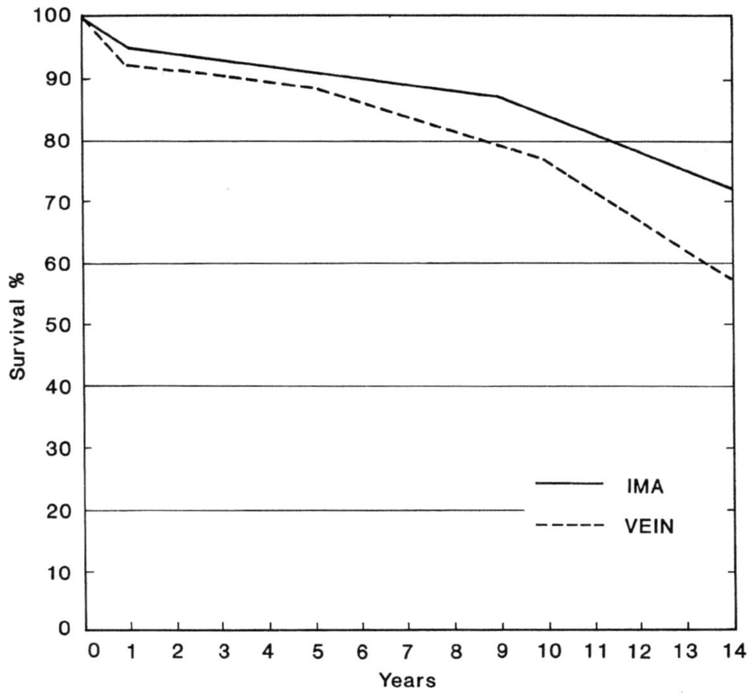

Fig. 106. Survival rates after internal mammary artery grafting in general compared to saphenous vein grafting (data compiled from the literature as shown in Table 4)

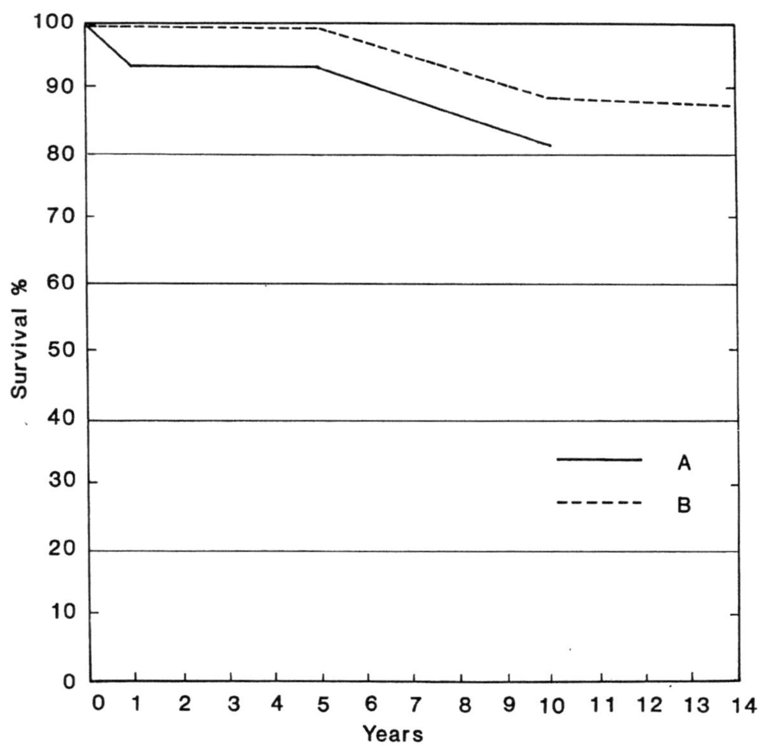

Fig. 107. Survival rates after expanded internal mammary artery grafting including sequential internal mammary artery grafts, bilateral internal mammary artery grafts and free internal mammary artery grafts: **A** data compiled from the literature as shown in Table 4; **B** Cameron et al. (1986)

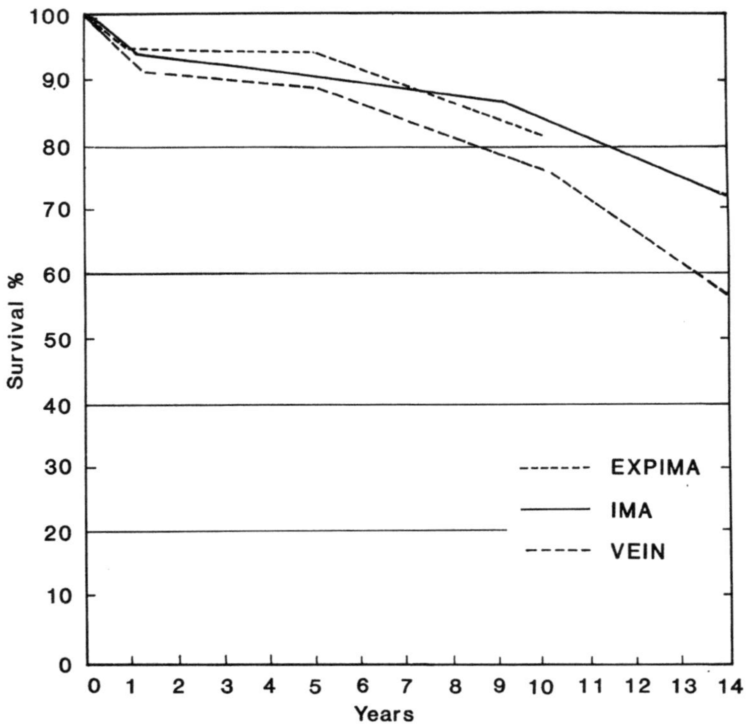

Fig. 108. Survival rates after expanded internal mammary artery grafting (EXPIMA) in comparison to unilateral internal mammary artery grafting (IMA) and saphenous VEIN grafting (data compiled from the literature as shown in Table 4)

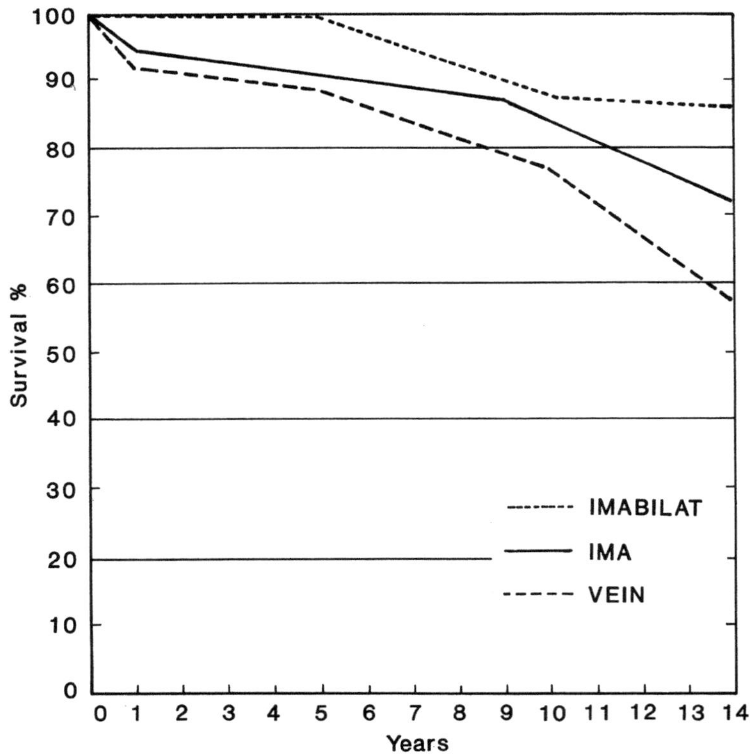

Fig. 109. Survival rates during 15 years of follow-up for bilateral internal mammary artery grafting (IMABILAT), unilateral internal mammary artery grafting (IMA), and saphenous VEIN grafting as reported by Cameron et al. (1986): complete data is available for 14 years.

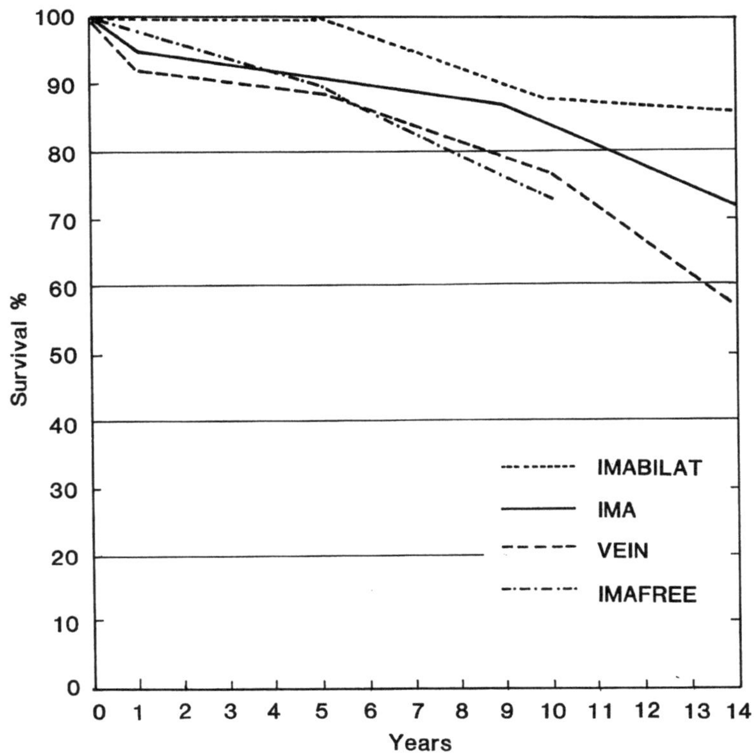

Fig. 110. Long-term survival rates after free internal mammary artery grafting (IMAFREE), saphenous VEIN grafting, unilateral internal mammary artery grafting (IMA), and bilateral internal mammary artery grafting (IMABILAT) (data compiled from the literature as shown in Table 4)

with respect to the early results. As mentioned by Loop et al. (1986b) this might be due to the delicate proximal anastomosis necessary for construction of the free internal mammary artery graft and the long-term results might improve after a learning curve as observed with other techniques. Only early and medium term results are actually available for sequential internal mammary artery grafts and therefore their place in optimal coronary artery revascularization is not clear yet.

9 Complications of Internal Mammary Artery Grafting

9.1 Inadequate Flow After Internal Mammary Artery–Coronary Artery Revascularization

The fact that the internal mammary artery is a living conduit with the capability of dilatation to meet increasing demand during exercise is combined with the risk of vasoconstriction. Vasoconstriction of an internal mammary artery graft (see Sect. 5.) can be fatal during periods of increased nutritional demand, such as weaning from cradiopulmonary bypass if not recognized in time. The experience with inadequate flow after internal mammary artery-coronary artery anastomoses was reported by von Segesser et al. in 1987[3].

9.1.1 Patients and Methods

Aortocoronary bypass surgery was performed in 250 consecutive patients over a period of 19 months between January 1985 and July 1986 at Geneva University Hospital. Mean age of the patients was 59 ± 9 years. A total of twenty procedures (8%) were redo revascularizations.

At least one internal mammary artery was used whenever possible. After standard internal mammary artery harvesting as a pedicle by low power electrocautery the patient was connected to cardiopulmonary bypass. Revascularization was performed under moderate hypothermia, cardioplegic arrest of the heart (high potassium, crystalloid), and intrapericardial cooling of the heart with cold saline. The distal anastomoses of the saphenous vein grafts were performed first. Internal mammary artery–coronary artery anastomoses were only performed if the flow was adequate.

[3] Reprinted with permission from the Thoracic and Cardiovascular Surgeon, Vol 35: 352–354, 1987

9.1.2 Results

There was at least one internal mammary artery–coronary artery anastomosis in 222 patients (89%). Multiple (bilateral, and/or sequential) internal mammary artery–coronary artery anastomoses were performed in 77 patients (31%). The revascularization of the coronary arteries was completed whenever necessary with saphenous vein grafts. The mean number of bypasses per patient was 2.8. Weaning from cardiopulmonary bypass was feasible in all but two patients (99.2%). Two other patients developed low cardiac output after decannulation, but still in the operating room. Of the four patients (1.6%) one had simple internal mammary artery- coronary artery anastomosis, and 3 of them had bilateral internal mammary artery–coronary artery anastomoses as shown in Table 5. Mean age in these patients was 54 ± 17 years and mean number of bypasses was 2.5.

As all four patients showed signs of left ventricular failure and left ventricular ischemia, they were connected again to cardiopulmonary bypass while a saphenous vein was harvested. An additional venous aorto–coronary bypass to the left anterior descending coronary artery, distal to the internal mammary artery–coronary artery anastomosis was constructed thereafter. All 4 patients showed evidence of patency of the internal mammary artery-coronary artery anastomosis as there was flow in the left anterior descending coronary artery originating from the left internal mammary artery as checked with a vascular clamp. Weaning from cardiopulmonary bypass was then possible in three of four patients. One patient with redo coronary artery revascularization could not be weaned from cardiopulmonary bypass despite the additional

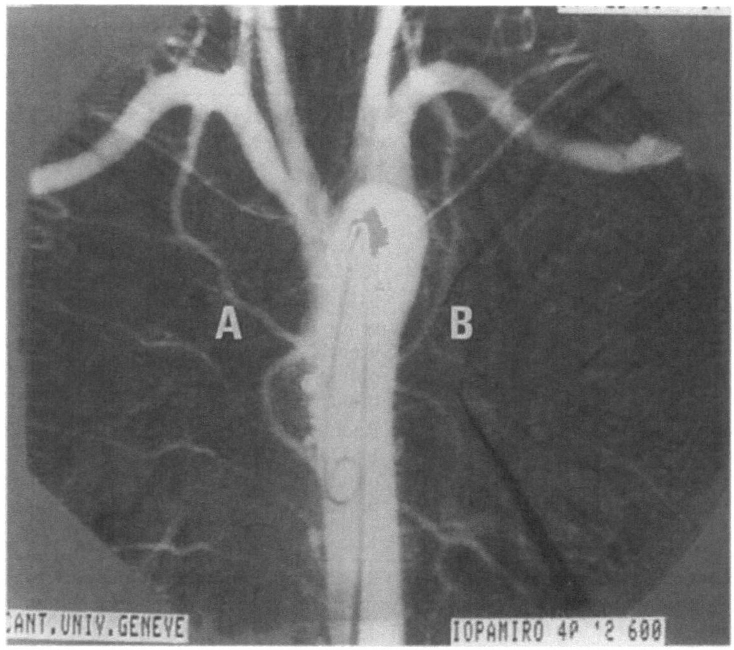

Fig. 111. Digital subtraction angiography showing patent right (**A**) and left (**B**) internal mammary artery graft as well as patent additional saphenous vein graft

saphenous vein graft and the use of the intra-aortic balloon pump (case 4). Overall in-hospital mortality was 6/250 patients or 2.4% including case 4. Digital subtraction angiography (DSA) showed patent bilateral internal mammary artery–coronary artery anastomoses as well as a patent additional vein graft at postoperative follow-up of case 1 (Fig. 111).

9.1.3 Comments

Internal mammary artery–coronary artery anastomoses provide inadequate nutritional support for the myocardium in some patients. In the present series 3/250 (1.2%) showed left ventricular failure and evidence of anterior ischemia during or shortly after weaning from cardiopulmonary bypass. They were successfully treated by immediate additional venous aortocoronary bypass onto the left anterior coronary artery already bypassed, with good early and medium-term results (see Table 5).

Inadequate nutritional support for the myocardium after internal mammary artery–coronary artery grafting can be due to internal mammary artery spasm, mismatch of the internal mammary artery in relation to the revascularized coronary arteries, residual stenosis in the recipient vessel, and technical problems at the site of the anastomosis or over the course of the internal mammary artery pedicle.

Spasms of the internal mammary artery are due to the fact, that this vessel is a living conduit which can increase and decrease its luminal diameter. Every cardiovascular surgeon using the internal mammary artery has observed poor or even absent flow in the transected internal mammary artery graft, which can be increased by vasodilators or mechanical manipulations. Furthermore, it has been shown that vasoactive drugs affect the flow in anastomosed internal mammary arteries (Jett et al. 1987).

Papaverine is therefore used topically by many surgeons and small but continuous systemical dose of nitrates and/or nifedipin is also advocated. In the present series topical and systemical medicamentous vasodilating techniques were used. But whether the final flow is sufficient or not is not decided by the surgeon, but by the myocardium. It is well known from the literature on coronary

Table 5. Inadequate flow after internal mammary artery–coronary artery anastomoses

No	Sex	Age (years)	NYHA	Operation	Additional bypass	Outcome
1	F	26	II	LIMA onto LAD, RIMA onto LCX	Vein onto LAD	Normal ejection fraction (scintigraphic), patent IMAs (angiographic)
2	M	56	III	LIMA onto LAD, RIMA onto LCX	Vein onto LAD	NYHA I at 6 months
3	M	71	III	LIMA onto LAD, vein onto diagonal branch, vein onto obtuse marginal branch	Vein onto LAD	NYHA I at 6 months
4	M	64	IV	Redo: LIMA onto LAD, RIMA onto obtuse marginal branch, vein onto RCA	Vein onto LAD, IABP	irreversible low output failure

LIMA left internal mammary artery; RIMA right internal mammary artery; LAD left anterior descending coronary artery; RCA right coronary artery; IABP intra-aortic balloon pump; NYHA New York Heart Association functional class

artery revascularization, that initial flow delivered by saphenous vein grafts is significantly higher than by internal mammary artery grafts. This has even been demonstrated for the same coronary artery bed, where vein flow was 2.7 times higher than internal mammary artery flow (Flemma et al. 1975). Mismatch of the internal mammary artery in relation to the revascularized coronary artery should be avoided. Absolute size of the internal mammary artery is less important as long as the internal mammary artery brings additional flow to the grafted coronary artery. If the internal mammary artery has to substitute a previously patent coronary artery or bypass however, as in revascularization after resection of coronary artery aneurysm (von Segesser et al. 1987c) or as in redo procedures with replacement of a moderately stenosed old saphenous vein graft, adequate size of the internal mammary artery graft is of prime importance .

Spasms, mismatch and technical problems of internal mammary artery grafts, either isolated or combined, lead to inadequate perfusion of the involved myocardium and eventually death if countermeasures are delayed. Immediate additional saphenous vein grafting onto the coronary artery already revascularized with an internal mammary artery graft, when ischemia persits, has proved to be the treatment of choice in these cases.

9.2 Spasms After Coronary Artery Revascularization

Spasms were reported for the coronary arteries by many authors as reviewed by Conti et al. (1979), can occur immediately (Buxton et al. 1981), or late after coronary artery revascularization (Singh and Varat 1982), and can also involve internal mammary artery grafts and/or coronary arteries as discussed in Sect. 9.1.

9.2.1 Coronary Artery Spasm Immediately After Saphenous Vein Grafting

Buxton et al. (1981) have investigated coronary artery spasm in six patients who had unexpected hemodynamic collapse within 2 h after cardiopulmonary bypass. All six had profound hypotension and recurrent ST segment elevation in electrocardiographic leads II,III, and aVF. All had either normal or noncritical luminal irregularities of dominant right coronary arteries and more than 75% occlusions of the left coronary circulation. Right coronary artery spasm, which was reversed after intracoronary nitroglycerin, was demonstrated angiographically in one patient; a patent right coronary artery was found at autopsy in another patient. Three patients died despite large intravenous doses of nitroglycerin. Two patients who had been unresponsive to intravenous nitroglycerin recovered after direct infusion of nitroglycerin into the right coronary artery. The authors concluded that coronary artery spasm immediately after myocardial revascularization may cause circulatory collapse and death; although the spasm may be refractory to usual therapy, it may respond to intracoronary nitroglycerin.

Significant increase in coronary arterial diameter has also been shown 20 s after intracoronary injection of papaverine (2 mg per cc of saline) into either the left (12 mg) or right (8 mg) coronary artery by coronary-artery cineangiograms (Carlson et al. 1988).

9.2.2 Spasm After Internal Mammary Artery Grafting

If spasms of the coronary arteries can occur immediately after saphenous vein grafting, there can be no doubt that spasm can also occur after internal mammary artery grafting. However, there are only a few reports in the literature (Pichard et al. 1980, Sarabu et al. 1987). Three mechanisms have to be considered:

1. Spasm of the internal mammary artery as documented in Sect. 5.1
2. Spasm of the coronary arteries as reported after saphenous vein grafts by Buxton et al. 1981
3. Spasm of the internal mammary artery grafts and the coronary arteries as a result of 1 or 2

Spasm of the internal mammary artery (1) can be treated either by indirect and/or direct application of vasodilating mediators and if insufficient by an additional saphenous vein graft as reported in Sect. 9.1. In the reported series, this approach was successful in 3/4 cases.

Spasm of the coronary arteries (2) after internal mammary artery grafting is more difficult to deal with as the coronary arteries can not be replaced with a passive vessel. If classical systemic application and direct intracoronary injection of vasoactive drugs fail to release the coronary artery spasm and a hypotensive status occurs due to low cardiac output it may be difficult to escape the vicious circle as consecutive internal mammary artery spasm may occur. The only way to reopen at least the internal mammary artery is to reperfuse the patient with the pump oxygenator and eventually to implant an additional passive vein graft. One has to remember here that driving pressure remains the main factor assuring adequat internal mammary artery flow (Beavis et al. 1988, von Segesser et al. 1989a).

Spasm of the internal mammary artery graft and the coronary arteries combined (3) are extremely difficult to deal with as pharmacological agents used to increase cardiac output may increase internal mammary artery spasm and therefore decrease coronary artery perfusion of already spastic coronary arteries.

If systemic and topical applications of vasodilators are without sufficient effect, and reperfusion and even additional passive vein grafts do not allow reversal of the spasm, the only remaining approach to save the patient is prolonged mechanical circulatory support.

9.3 Mechanical Circulatory Support After Internal Mammary Coronary Artery Grafting

Postcardiotomy patients with irreversible low cardiac output are a difficult subset of patients for mechanical circulatory support. In some patients with moderate pump failure, in whom reperfusion can be achieved with the pump oxygenator, the intra-aortic balloon pump may provide, in conjunction with positive inotropic medication and afterload reduction, the necessary minimal increase of myocardial perfusion for weaning and maybe even for recovery. In most reported series, there were some cases that could be saved with this approach.

There is another group of patients however, who will not respond to this treatment, but may eventually be saved by more invasive mechanical circulatory support, i.e., uni- or biventricular assist with artificial ventricles, either till recovery or transplantation. We have used this approach in some cases and report here one redo coronary artery revascularization procedure where a patient with coronary artery spasm could not be weaned from cardiopulmonary bypass despite all other technical and pharmacological measures including the intra-aortic balloon pump. Left ventricular assist by the means of a pneumatic paracorporeal ventricle (Abiomed) was installed in this patient and initially activated for maximal flow with an intra-aortic balloon-pump console (Fig. 112) as previously reported (von Segesser et al. 1988a, von Segesser L and Turina M, 1990). Left ventricular ejection fraction was monitored with bidimensional echocardiography and weaning from the left ventricular assist device was started successfully at the 7th postoperative day. The patient recovered and had a final left ventricular ejection fraction > 30% in comparison to 0% at the first postoperative day. This experience shows, that invasive mechanical circulatory support can be promising in selected cases with postcardiotomy pump failure after internal mammary artery-coronary artery grafting.

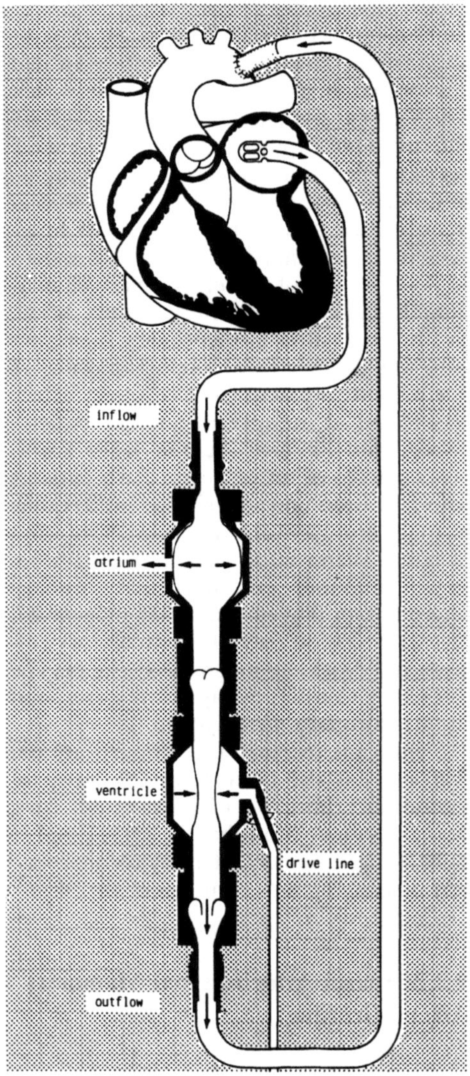

Fig. 112. Paracorporeal ventricle assist device including atrium, ventricle, and two tricuspid valves (Abiomed)

9.4 Sternal Infections Following Internal Mammary Artery – Coronary Artery Grafting

Although complications associated with median sternotomy are usually infrequent, numerous reports in the literature describe the increased morbidity and mortality when median sternotomy is followed by sternal dehiscence, osteomyelitis, or chronic chondritis. Culliford et al. (1976) have analyzed a series 39 sternal or costochondral infections from a series of 2594 cases with open-heart surgery. Most of these infections were associated with a number of presdisposing factors: prolonged perfusion time, excessive postoperative bleeding, depressed cardiac output in the postoperative period, and a history of reexploration for the control of hemorrhage.

As previously reported (von Segesser et al. 1986a) there was no significant difference in rethoracotomy rate for control of hemorrhage in a series of 100 procedures with internal mammary artery grafting (5%) in comparison to a series of 250 procedures with saphenous vein grafting (5%). However, there is increasing concern about sternal infections following internal mammary artery-coronary artery grafting because of the potential devascularization due to the take-down procedure.

Nkongho et al. (1984) have studied the question of sternotomy infection after harvesting of the internal mammary artery. In their experience (483 consecutive patients), the use of the internal mammary artery did not significantly increase the incidence of postoperative median sternotomy infection: solely vein grafting 1/226 (0.5%), unilateral internal mammary artery grafting 2/149 (1.3%), other procedures with cardiopulmonary bypass 3/108 (2.8%). But when infection does occur in patients with internal mammary artery grafting, successful treatment is more likely to require more aggressive surgical manipulation, such as the use of vascularized muscle pedicle grafts, to eventually close the sternal defect.

In the series of Cosgrove et al. (1988), wound complications were more common in patients with bilateral internal mammary artery grafts than in those with saphenous vein grafts or receiving single internal mammary artery grafts. There were no complications in patients receiving only saphenous vein grafts, 1/338 (0.3%) in patients receiving one internal mammary artery graft and 8/338 (2.3%) in patients receiving two internal mammary artery grafts (**P** < 0.002). The prevalence of wound complications in patients with diabetes mellitus was 5.7% and in those without diabetes mellitus, 0.3% (**P** < 0.01). The prevalence of wound complications in patients less than 60 years of age was 0.2%, in patients in their 60 s, 1.6%, and in patients older than 70, 3.1% (**P** < 0.01). Multivariate logistic regression analysis identified diabetes mellitus and age, but not bilateral internal mammary artery grafting as risk factors for wound complications.

Our current approach for sternotomy infection after internal mammary artery grafting includes thorough debridement, implantation of chains of gentamicin beads (von Segesser et al. 1988), and rewiring. If this treatment fails repeatedly, the use of vascularized muscle pedicle grafts may be indicated as reported in Sect. 8.1.1.

9.5 Other Complications After Internal Mammary Artery Grafting

Complications of internal mammary artery-coronary artery grafting were reported by Olearchyk and Magovern (1986) for a series of 833 patients who were operated upon between 1968 and 1981. In their series the most common complication was perioperative infarction, which occurred in 61 (7.3%) patients. Atrial flutter or fibrillation was detected in 36 (4.3%) and right or left bundle branch block with or without second- or third-degree atrioventricular block was observed in 32 (3.8%). Mediastinal exploration for bleeding was necessary in 24 (2.9%) patients; 19 (2.3%) patients had debridement and closure of sternal dehiscence. Deep venous thrombosis and pulmonary embolism developed in 10 patients (1.2%); 2 patients died after stroke. Tearing of the ascending aorta because of application of a partial occlusion clamp, development of a left internal mammary artery graft–pulmonary artery fistula, peripheral thromboembolism, and phrenic nerve injury occurred in one patient each.

Further reported complications include kinking of internal mammary artery grafts (Brenot et al. 1988), pulmonary effects of pleurotomy (Burgess et al. 1978), phrenic paresis (Wilcox et al. 1988), upper rib fractures with potential brachial plexus injury (Woodring et al. 1985), chylothorax (Zakhour et al. 1988, Di Summa et al. 1988), coronary – subclavian steal from reversed flow in the internal mammary artery used for coronary bypass (Valentine et al. 1987, Marshall et al. 1988, Olson et al. 1988), residual pain after myocardial revascularization with the internal mammary artery due to anomalous origin of the left thyreocervical trunk (Tartini et al. 1984) and leg ischemia (Adar et al. 1988).

10 Long Term Follow-up After Internal Mammary Artery–Coronary Artery Revascularization

Long-term survival based on the figures reported in the literature is shown Table 4; curves are plotted in Sect. 8.3. Late results of internal mammary artery–coronary artery grafting are derived from this data pool and may give a general impression of the available long-term results. However, studies with complete follow-up are exceptional, and therefore the results given have to be interpreted with care. Some techniques may appear superior due to the nonrandom selection of patients. Objective assessment of graft patency rates in larger series of operated patients that are complete over longer periods of time, still do not exist.

10.1 Freedom from Reinfarction After Coronary Artery Revascularization

Time to first new myocardial infarction in patients in the registry of the Coronary Artery Surgery Study (CASS) with severe angina and three vessel disease, comparing medical and early surgical therapy, was studied by Myers et al. (1988) during a 6-year follow-up. There were 679 medically treated patients and 1921 surgically treated patients in that nonrandomized comparison. A broad definition of myocardial infarction incorporating electrocardiographic and clinical criteria was used to include as many new infarctions as possible. Patients were stratified by left ventricular wall motion score and number of proximal coronary artery stenoses; after adjustment for these variables, 86% of surgical and 73% of medical patients were free of new myocardial infarction at 6 years (**P** < 0.0001). This advantage of surgical treatment was observed in subgroups of patients with at least one proximal 70% (or greater) stenosis in the left anterior descending coronary artery and moderate or severe impairment of left ventricular function, as well as those patients with two proximal coronary artery narrowings. In a multivariate (Cox) analysis of preoperative clinical, hemodynamic, and angiographic factors, early operation was the strongest predictor of freedom from new myocardial infarction. Fatal myocardial infarction occurred in 9.3% of the medical group and in 2.0% of the surgical group (**P** < 0.001). Although the authors could not control for all possible biases in this nonrandomized comparison, the reported data strongly support the inference that direct coronary revascularization lowers the incidence of and fatalities from subsequent myocardial infarction in subsets of patients with severe preoperative angina pectoris and three-vessel coronary artery disease.

The results of this study were obtained in a period when coronary artery revascularization was mainly performed with saphenous vein grafts. In the meanwhile, coronary artery surgery has progressed and even better results might be achieved nowadays. However, the final proof of substantial benefit due to coronary artery revascularization can only be achieved if graft patency has been demonstrated.

10.2 Objective Assessment of the Results of Internal Mammary Artery–Coronary Artery Revascularization

Many noninvasive and invasive techniques have been developed for subjective and objective assessment of the results of coronary artery revascularization. The most frequently used include assessment of New York Heart Association functional status, return to work, ergometry, echocardiography, scintigraphy, angiography. Other more recent techniques, such as magnetic resonance imaging (MR) and positron emission tomography (PET) are still in development.

At our institution a routine control with ergometry is scheduled three months after operation for all patients undergoing heart surgery. More invasive procedures are performed in patients with New York Heart Association functional class > 1, positive ergometry, or who did not resume work.

10.2.1 Scintigraphic Evaluation

Scintigraphic studies of the myocardium before and after myocardial revasculariaztion allow the analysis of normal, ischemic or scarred myocardium, as well as determination of left ventricular ejection fraction including stress test for functional analysis. Classic techniques include thallium and technetium pyrophosphate studies. However new radiopharmaceuticals with higher photon flow and shorter half-life are available now. Figure 113 shows a myocardial scintigraphic image obtained with a technetium radiopharmaceutical which also allows to realize myocardial single-photon emission computerized tomography, better known as SPECT.

In symptomatic patients, either due to impaired ventricular function or angina, the differentiation between scarred myocardial segments and ischemic myocardial segments is of prime importance, as the latter can potentially be revascularized. The decision for an eventual redo revascularization, either by the invasive cardiologist or by the surgeon, however, has to be evaluated individually as a function of the anatomic situation, the myocardial area at risk, and the patient's general condition.

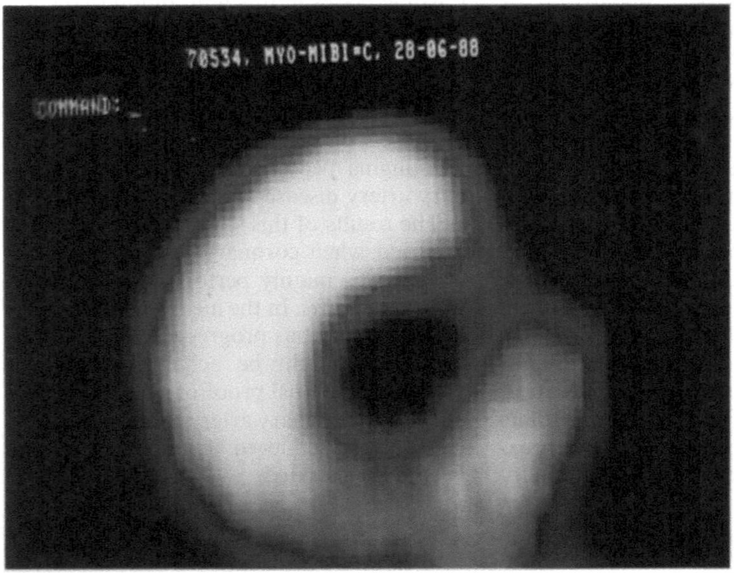

Fig. 113. $^{99}Tc^{m}$ scintigraphy of a left ventricular section showing hypoperfusion of the posterior wall

10.2.2 Angiographic Evaluation

Angiographic evaluation of coronary artery grafts can be performed by digital subtraction angiography as shown in Fig. 111. Steffenino et al. (1985) have shown that nonselective, intra-arterial, electrocardiogram-triggered digital subtraction angiography can visualize patent saphenous vein grafts with a high sensitivity and may be a useful screening tool for bypass graft patency; false negatives, however, and poor visualization of distal anastomoses limit its routine use and direct dye injection into the grafts during coronary angiography is required for precise analysis. Two projections are in general necessary to assess the three-dimensional quality of a graft as demonstrated for a saphenous vein graft in Figs 114 and 115.

Demonstration of internal mammary artery grafts, their anastomoses and the distal coronary artery bed is somewhat more delicate.

A left internal mammary artery graft revascularizing the left anterior descending coronary artery by an end-to-side anastomosis is shown in Fig. 116. Figures 117 and 118 show the pictures obtained from a sequential left internal mammary artery graft revascularizing side-to-side the diagonal branch and end-to-side the left anterior descending coronary artery.

If stenoses over the course of saphenous vein grafts are increasingly frequent with time (see Figs 1 and 2), these lesions are exceptional with internal mammary artery grafts. In cases with reduced flow in internal mammary artery grafts due to stenosis this is in general situated at the level of the internal mammary artery–coronary artery anastomosis (Fig. 119) or in the distal coronary artery bed. In situations where a saphenous vein graft would occlude because of low flow, the internal mammary artery may remain patent for years over its entire length (Fig. 120) due to the minimal circulation by

Fig. 114. Saphenous vein graft visualized by direct dye injection 8 years after implantation onto the left anterior descending coronary artery: severe luminal narrowing

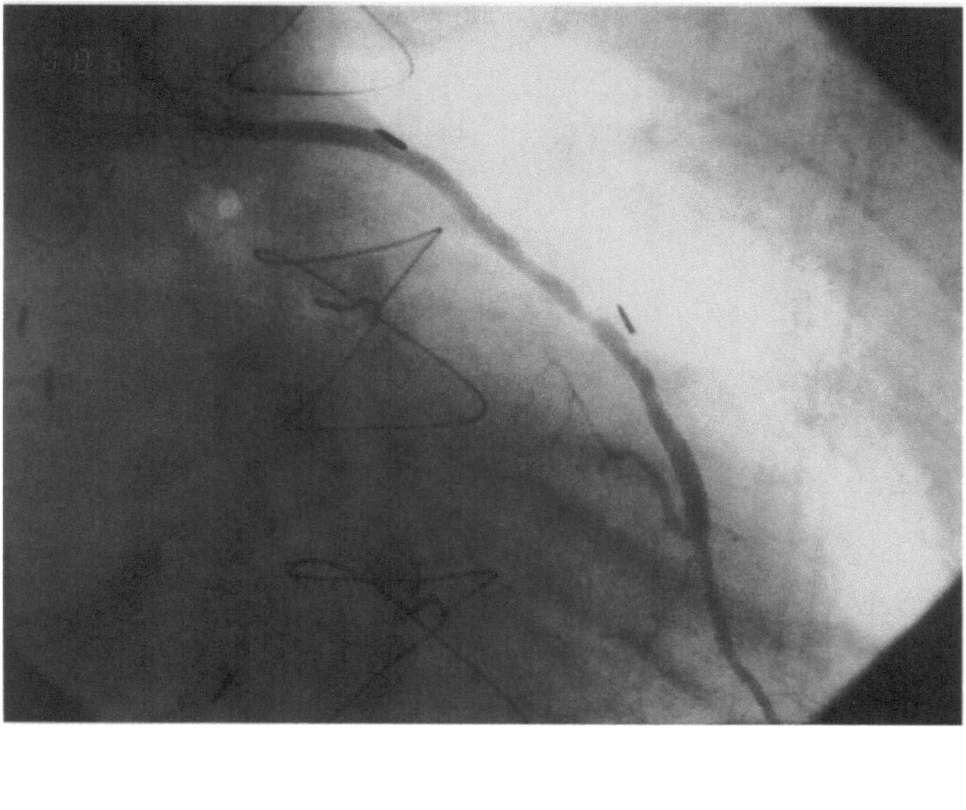

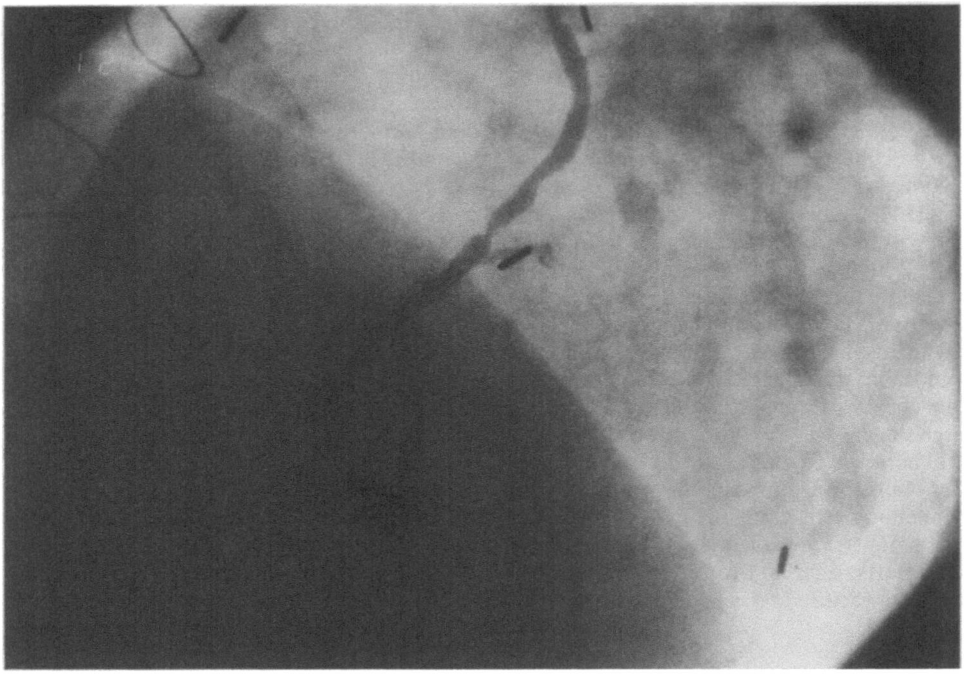

Fig. 115. Second plane of the saphenous vein graft shown in Fig. 114: severe luminal narrowing is confirmed

Fig. 116. Direct angiogram of a left internal mammary artery revascularizing the left anterior coronary artery by an end-to-side anastomosis

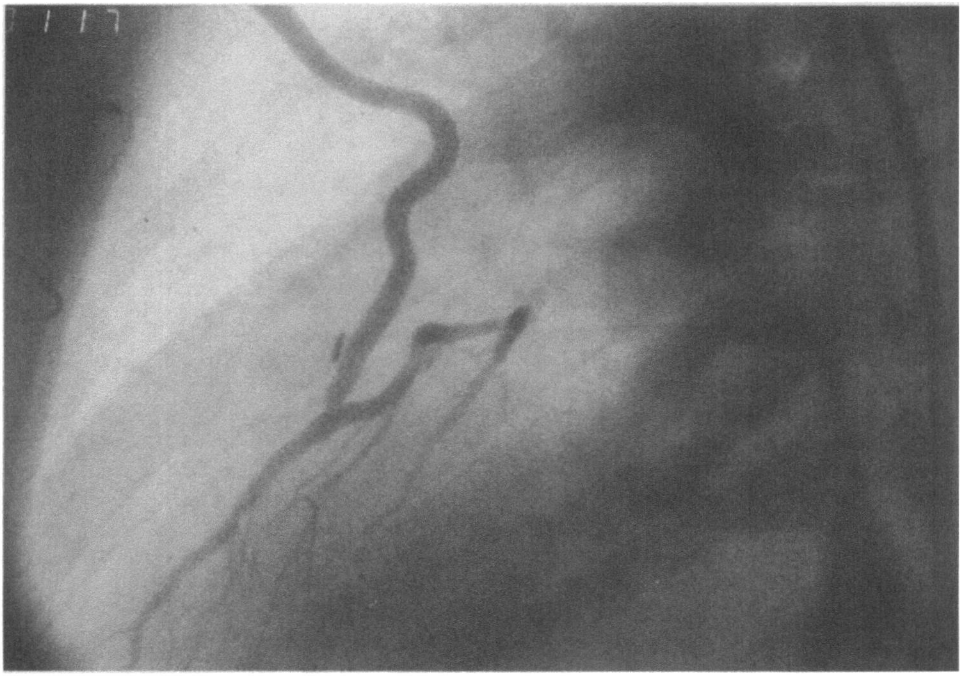

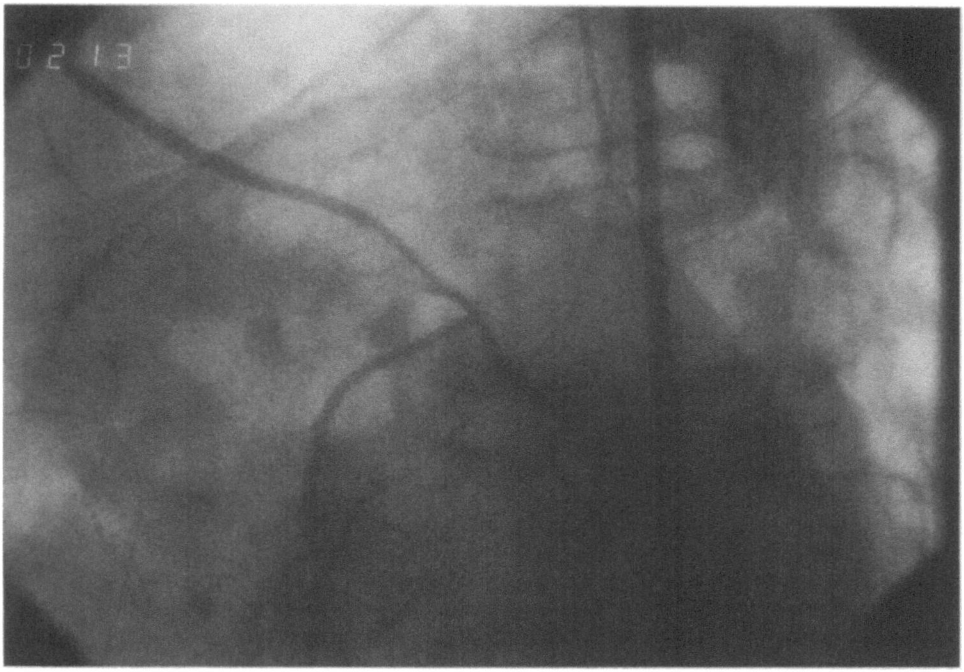

Fig. 117. Direct angiogram of sequential left internal mammary artery revascularizing the diagonal branch by a side-to-side anastomosis and the left anterior descending coronary artery by an end-to-side anastomosis

Fig. 118. Indirect angiogram of a sequential left internal mammary artery graft revascularizing the diagonal branch by a side-to-side anastomosis and the left anterior descending coronary artery by an end-to-side anastomosis

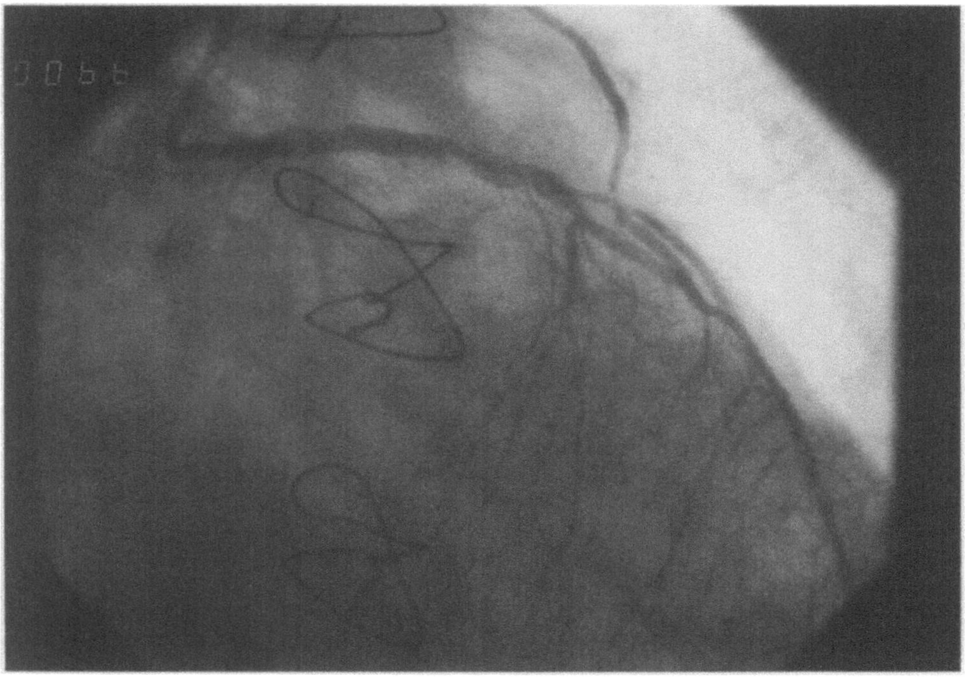

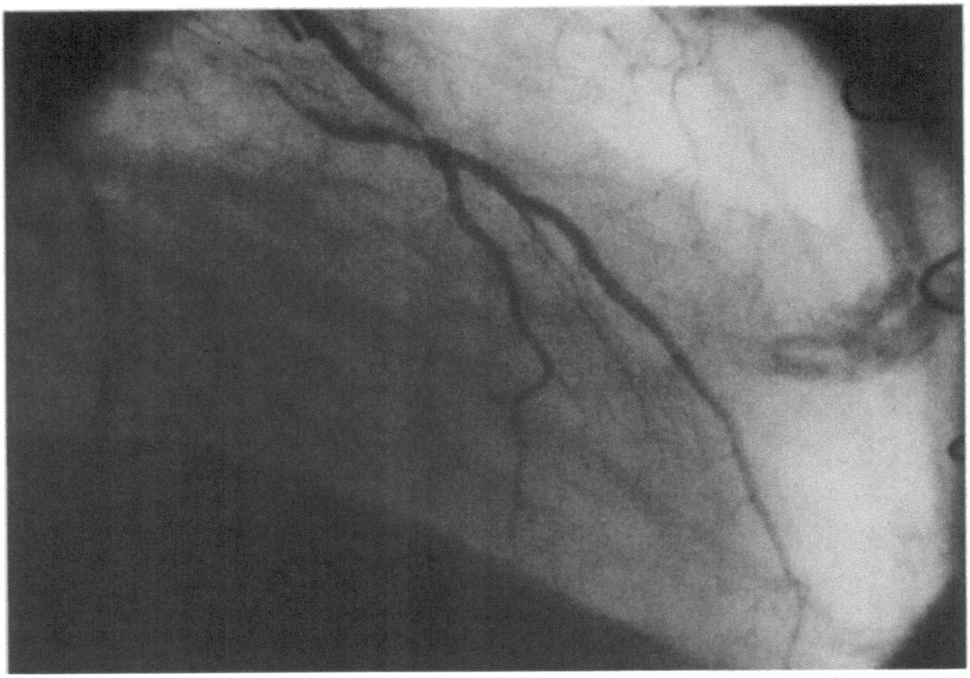

Fig. 119. Direct angiogram of a left internal mammary artery graft with stenosis at the anastomotic site to the left anterior descending coronary artery

Fig. 120. Direct angiogram of an internal mammary artery graft with occlusion of the internal mammary artery–coronary artery anastomosis: dye progresses faster in collaterals (**A**) than in the internal mammary artery (**B**)

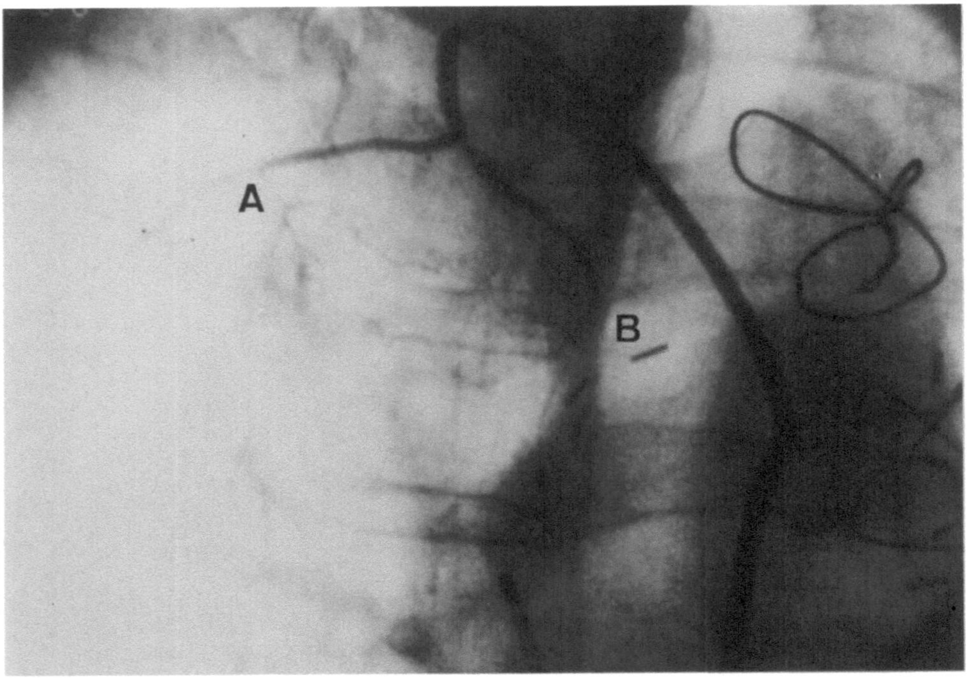

microanastomoses with surrounding tissue and within its pedicle similar to the Vineberg procedure. Furthermore, restoration of patency after apparent occlusion associated with progression of coronary artery disease has also been reported (Dincer and Barner 1983).

10.3 Late Patency Rates of Internal Mammary Artery Grafts

Patency rates in clinical internal mammary artery–coronary artery grafting has been reported in several studies over the last 15 years. It is however difficult to get an overall impression of the very disparate results in the various studies. The available patency rates of coronary artery grafts, assessed by angiography, including internal mammary artery grafts and saphenous vein grafts reported in the literature are shown in Table 6. Early patency at 30 days varies between 100% and 84% for internal mammary artery grafts and 92% and 70% for saphenous vein grafts depending on the study selected. Mean values ± standard deviation of patency rates for the various types of grafts at different intervals have been calculated for this data pool, summerizing the results of far more than 10 000 coronary artery revascularization procedures. Patency rates for left internal mammary artery–left anterior descending coronary artery are best documented: mean patency rate is 91.8% ± 4.5% after 1 month (8 reports), 92.3% ± 5.6% after 1 year (7 reports), 81.0% ± 20.2% after 5 years (5 reports), and 71.6% ± 20.1% after 10 years (3 reports). The fact that the data for different intervals arise from different studies is responsible for the apparent increase in patency between between the first month and the first year. Despite the report of Aris et al. (1987), on isolated cases with initial internal mammary artery graft "occlusion" and no flow, overall graft patency decreases with time, and the figures shown represent the data compiled in the literature over a 15-year period, with more early results than late results, and improved results in more recent studies.

The results for internal mammary artery grafts in general are as follows: 93.2% ± 4.5% at 1 year (6 studies), 91.6% ± 3.2% after 5 years (3 studies), and 63.5% ± 17.7% after 10 years (2 studies). As expected, patency rates for left internal mammary artery grafting onto the left anterior descending coronary artery are somewhat better at 10 years in comparison to internal mammary artery grafting in general (Fig. 121) as also shown in individual studies analyzing this point (Huddlestone et al. 1986). The present variations are again due to the different subsets of studies analyzed at different intervals. These results however represent the reported analyses and have to be compared to the patency rates obtained with saphenous vein grafting: 84.8% ± 4.6% after 1 year (8 studies), 70.8% ± 8.4% after 5 years (4 studies), and 55.2% ± 21.1% after 10 years (6 studies) as shown in Figs. 122 and 123. The patency rates of internal mammary artery grafts were far superior in all long-term studies comparing them to saphenous vein grafts. However, these results have to be interpreted with care, as the mean restudy rate is only 53.2% ± 32.3% (range 6%-100%) in 50 reported subsets of patients where the restudy rate could be assessed from the available data. To the best of our knowledge, there are only two reports with 100% follow-up of the grafts studied (Barner et al. 1974: **n** = 150, Singh et al. 1983: **n** = 33). In many studies the proportion of restudied grafts cannot even be assessed (18 reported subsets).

A unique randomized prospective study with 10-year follow-up comparing internal mammary artery grafts (**n** = 39) versus saphenous vein grafts (**n** = 41) for revascularization of the left anterior descending coronary artery was reported by Zeff et al.(1988). Overall followup rate was 97.5% in their series. They reported 10-year survival of 92.3% for internal mammary artery grafts and 82.1% for saphenous vein grafts. At catheterization after a mean interval of more than 8.6 years, the mean patency rate for internal mammary artery grafts was 94.6% versus 76.3% for saphenous vein grafts (**P** < 0.01). The authors

Table 6. Patency rates

Reference	Type of graft and vessel	Follow-up (mean)	No. of patients	Follow-up rate (%)	Patency rate (%)
Loop et al. 1973	LIMA–LAD, CX	10 months	100	65	97
	Veins	10 months	100	65	85
Kay et al. 1974	IMA–LAD, LCX, RCA	20 months	628	15	99
	Veins	20 months	628	15	84
Barner 1974a	LIMA	7 days	100	90	97
		1 year		22	100
	RIMA	7 days		90	95
		1 year		23	96
Grondin et al. 1975	Veins	14 days	100	88	92
		1 year		71	85
	IMA	14 days	40	93	97
		1 year		84	88
Barner et al. 1976	RIMA	20 days	76	100	97
		13 months		100	95
	LIMA	20 days	139	100	90
		13 months		100	90
Green et al. 1979	IMA	> 1 year	121	26	92
	Veins	> 1 year	121	26	83
Lytle et al. 1980	LIMA–LAD	22 months	100	46	91
	Vein–LAD	20 months	100	56	79
Tyras et al. 1980	LIMA–LAD	30 days	765	69	84
		5 years		63	47
	Vein–LAD	30 days	694	69	70
		5 years		63	13
Chassignolle et al. 1982	LIMA–LAD	30 days	350	21	96
		> 4 years		6	100
Singh et al. 1983	IMA	3.6 years	33	100	93
	Veins	3.6 years	33	100	63
Speiser et al. 1983	LIMA–LAD	3 months	29	100	100
	Veins–LAD	3 months	29	100	86
Tector et al. 1983	IMA	< 2 years	298	14	93
		> 2 years	298	9	96
		> 6 years	298	6	94
Frey et al. 1984	Veins	1 year	82	<90	83
		9 years	55	?	65
Grondin et al. 1984	IMA	1 year	40	90	89
		10 years	40	50	76
	Veins	1 year	238	83	84
		10 years	238	24	53
Harjola et al. 1984	IMA sequential	5 years	61	?	98
		10 years	61	?	96
	Veins	5 years	61	?	78
		10 years	61	?	68
Okies et al. 1984	LIMA–LAD	30 days	259	?	96
		5 years		?	81
		10 years		?	69
	Vein–LAD	30 days	139	?	92
		5 years		?	64
		10 years			45

Table 6. (Continued)

Reference	Type of graft and vessel	Follow-up (mean)	No. of patients	Follow-up rate (%)	Patency rate (%)
Kamath et al.	Expanded IMA	21 months	87	41	93
1985	Veins	21 months	87	42	90
Huddlestone	IMA	1 year	4140	20	98
et al. 1986		5 years	4140	?	88
		10 years	4140	?	51
	Veins	1 year	4140	20	95
		5 years	4140	?	78
		10 years	4140	?	20
	LIMA	5 years	x/4140	?	89
		10 years	x/4140	?	53
	RIMA	5 years	4140−x	?	79
		10 years	4140−x	?	31
Loop et al.	LIMA–LAD	10 years	2306	37	93
1986a	Veins	10 years	3625	40	80
Loop et al. 1986b	Free IMA	49 months	256	26	77
Olearchyk and	LIMA–LAD	19 month	833	37	88
Magovern 1986	Veins	19 months	833	37	63
Rankin et al.	Expanded IMA	< 8 months	207	85	99
1986	Veins	< 8 months	207	85	91
Tector et al.	Expanded IMA	?	100	8	93
1986	Veins	?	100	8	80
Ivert et al. 1988	IMA	12 months	101	88	90
		5 years	80	75	89
		11 years	60	54	87
	Veins	12 months	61	88	83
		5 years	48	75	79
		11 years	33	54	60
Kuttler et al. 1988	IMA	7 days	166	45	96
Zeff et al.	LIMA–LAD	8.9 years	39	95	95
1988	Veins–LAD	8.6 years	41	76	76

The tabulated figures were calculated from the available data in the studies cited. However, indications, surgical techniques and data analyses may differ from one study to another
IMA internal mammary artery; LIMA left internal mammary artery; RIMA right internal mammary artery; unilat unilateral; bilat bilateral; sequent sequential anastomoses; LAD left anterior descending coronary artery; ? actual percentage of visualized grafts could not be assessed (in general actuarial analyses)

concluded that the left internal mammary artery is the conduit of choice for revascularization of the left anterior descending coronary artery.

Patency rates of expanded internal mammary artery grafting, defined as more than one internal mammary artery anastomosis (sequential internal mammary artery grafts, bilateral internal mammary artery grafts, and/or free internal mammary artery grafts) were also compiled from Table 6 and showed the following results: 99.0% patency at 1 year, 93.0% at 2 years and 88.8% ±11.0% at 4 years (Fig. 124). These patency rates are superior in comparison to saphenous vein grafts; however, they do not reach the results of unilateral internal mammary artery grafts after 4 years of follow up.

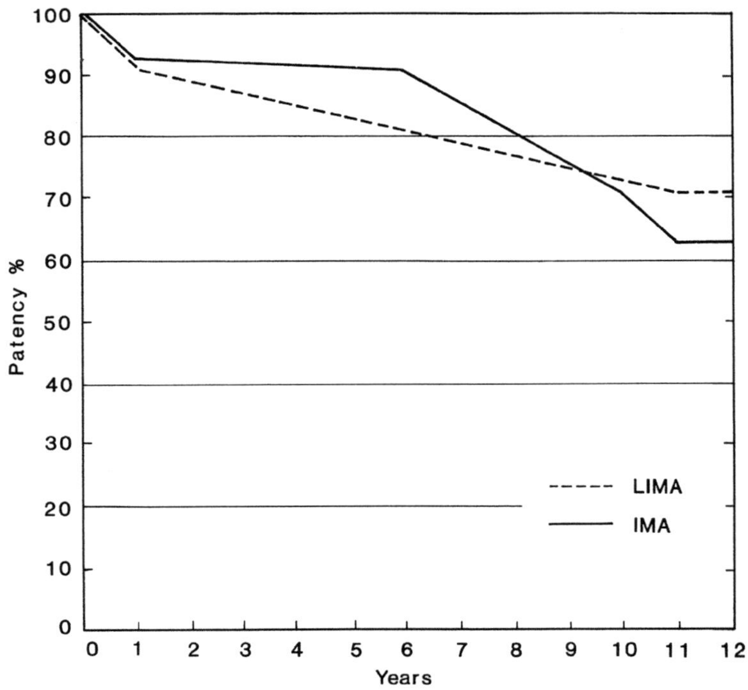

Fig. 121. Patency rates of left internal mammary artery grafts onto the left anterior descending coronary artery (LIMA) in comparison to internal mammary artery grafts (IMA) (data compiled from the literature as shown in Table 6)

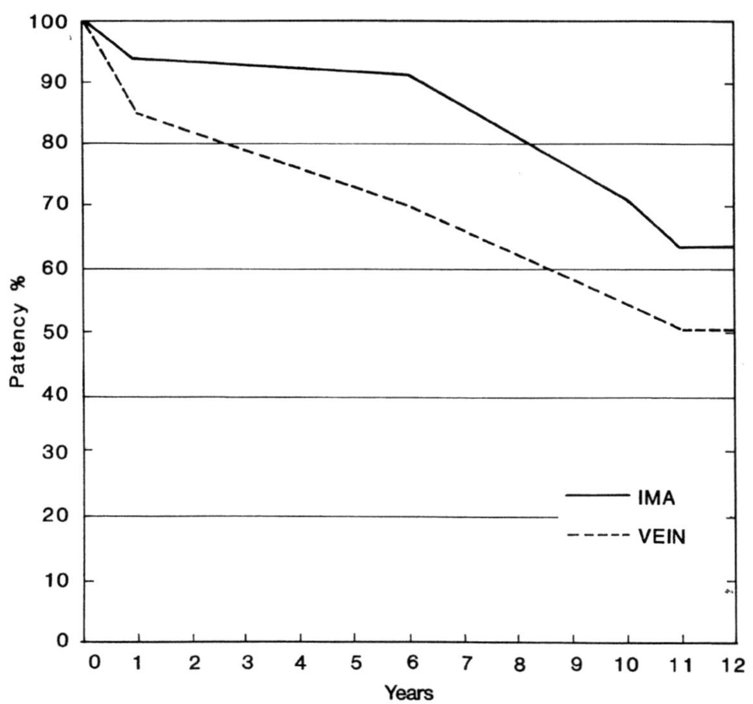

Fig. 122. Patency rates of internal mammary artery grafts in general (IMA) compared to saphenous VEIN grafts (data compiled from the literature as shown in Table 6)

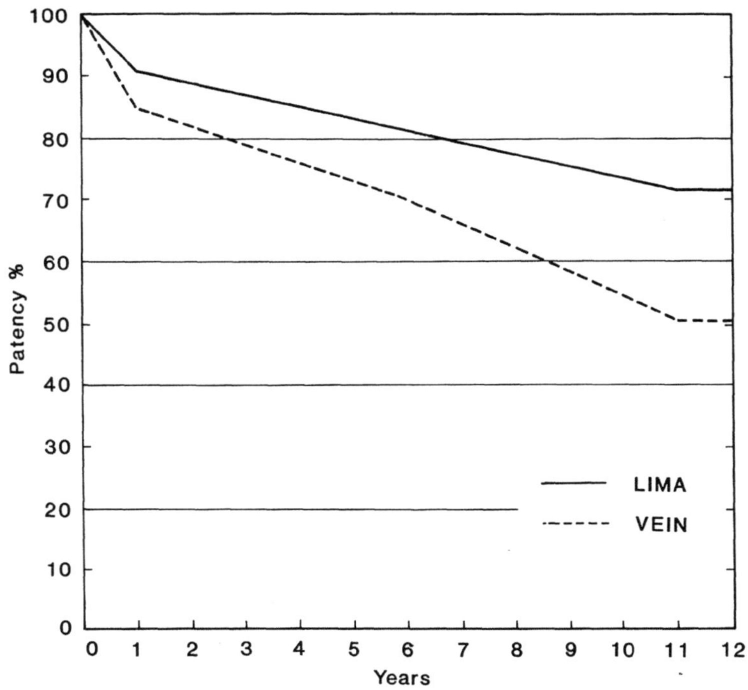

Fig. 123. Patency rates of left internal mammary artery grafts onto the left anterior descending coronary artery (LIMA) in comparison to saphenous VEIN grafts (data compiled from the literature as shown in Table 6)

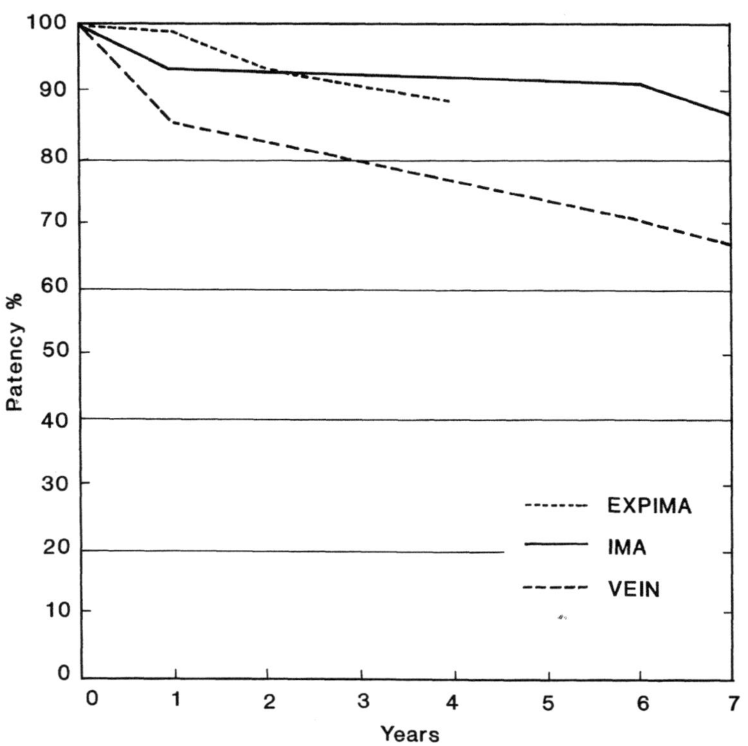

Fig. 124. Patency rates of expanded internal mammary artery grafting including sequential internal mammary artery grafts, bilateral internal mammary artery grafts, and free internal mammary artery grafts (EXPIMA) in comparison to left internal mammary artery grafts (LIMA) and saphenous VEIN grafts (data compiled from the literature as shown in Table 6)

11 Redo Coronary Artery Revascularization After Internal Mammary Artery Grafting

Coronary artery bypass grafts using the internal mammary artery as conduit have shown superior patency rates as compared to grafts made from saphenous veins (see Sect. 10.3) and other materials (see Sect. 5.4). Stenoses of internal mammary artery grafts, however, may occur in as many as 9% of patients within 22 months of implantation as reported by Lytle et al.(1980). Furthermore, attrition of saphenous vein grafts implanted for complementary revascularization (see Sect. 2.3), deterioration of the distal coronary bed of grafted vessels, as well as increasing arteriosclerosis of non-grafted vessels may require redo coronary artery revascularization after internal mammary artery grafting.

The indication as well as the type of procedure for redo coronary artery revascularization has to be evaluated individually as a function of the myocardium at risk, coronary anatomy, available bypass material, complexity of the revascularization procedure (associated valvular or congenital heart disease), and the patient's general condition. There is an increased risk of morbidity and mortality for redo revascularization procedures in comparison to primary coronary artery revascularizations for both percutaneous transluminal angioplasty and surgical revascularization. For the latter approach, Cameron et al. (1988) reported less early relief of angina than at initial operation. Therefore, careful analysis of each individual case is of prime importance for optimal results in this difficult subset of patients.

11.1 Percutaneous Transluminal Angioplasty After Internal Mammary Artery Grafting

Percutaneous transluminal angioplasty has been reported by Keriakes et al. (1985) for left internal mammary artery grafts and by Steffenino et al. (1986) for left and right internal mammary artery grafts. Angioplasties of the distal insertion of the internal mammary artery grafts and/or of the recipient vessels distal to them was performed and symptomatic improvement was obtained, illustrating the feasibility and safety of transluminal angioplasty of right and left internal mammary artery grafts, using the internal mammary artery as way of access. In other cases angioplasty of the proxymal native coronary artery bed was performed under "standby" of the internal mammary artery revascularizing the distal coronary artery bed of the same major coronary artery.

Allthough these techniques are available today, one has however to remember, that spastic reaction of the internal mammary artery can occur during manipulation, reducing the already inadequate coronary artery perfusion and also that surgical standby during the angioplasty procedure cannot provide similar safety as in previously non-operated patients because of the more complex redosternotomy and its potential complications.

11.2 Reoperation After Internal Mammary Artery Grafting

According to Fox et al. (1987), it is estimated that as many as 7% of patients who have an aortocoronary bypass operation will require a second bypass procedure within 10–12 years.

The morbidity and mortality of reoperation for coronary artery disease has been analyzed by Schaff et al.(1983). To determine late survival and functional status after second revascularization procedures for coronary artery disease, the authors studied 106 consecutive reoperated patients. Recurrence of angina was most commonly caused by bypass graft occlusion alone and in combination with progressive disease of the coronary arteries (60 patients, 57%). A total of 3 patients (2.8%) died within thirty days of reoperation; each death resulted from myocardial infarction. Actuarial survival of patients discharged alive was 94% at 5 years and 89% at 7 years. When recurrence of angina, the need of a third operation, and myocardial infarction are included with cardiac related deaths, eventfree survival is 28% at 5 years and 26% at 7 years. These results are clearly inferior to primary coronary artery revascularization.

A more recent series of 1500 coronary artery revascularizations reported by Lytle et al. (1987) showed a risk of death of 3.4% and a risk of myocardial infarction of 8% as compared to 1.0% and 0.6%, respectively for primary coronary artery revascularizations during the same time frame. The reasons for increased morbidity and mortality in redo procedures include suboptimal myocardial protection, less often "complete" revascularization, and eventually embolization of debris from atherosclerotic vein grafts.

The statement, that internal mammary artery grafts are superior to saphenous vein grafts also means that the former will deteriorate somewhat later. Together with the ongoing coronary artery sclerosis and the inherent attrition of saphenous vein grafts placed for complementary revascularization there will be sooner or later a considerable group of patients requiring reoperation after internal mammary artery grafting. Three situations in redo coronary artery revascularization after internal mammary artery grafting have to be distinguished.

11.2.1 Completely Occluded Internal Mammary Artery Graft

In this case, the reoperation procedure is like the procedure after saphenous vein grafting. The recommended strategies to adjust for the anatomic complexity of myocardial blood supply in reoperative patients include minimal dissection before aortic cross-clamping, low pressure infusion of cardioplegic solution into the aortic root, early disconnection of atherosclerotic grafts to avoid embolization of atherosclerotic material into the distal coronary arteries, perfusion of cardioplegic solution through new vein grafts, and deep hypothermia. The major problem in this situation may be to find an adequate amount of new graft material, suitable for coronary artery revascularization. Some coronary arteries can be revascularized by branches of the celiac trunk (see also Sect.5.4.1).

11.2.2 Patent, but Stenosed Internal Mammary Artery Graft

In this situation transection of the internal mammary artery graft with the oscillating saw or later during control for temporary clamping, should be avoided in order to be able to reuse the internal mammary artery graft. To provide adequate length for construction of a new anastomosis in general distally to the previous anastomosis, the internal mammary artery graft has to be mobilized as a reduced pedicle or as a naked graft. This dissection is tedious and there is a permanent risk of damaging the graft. Deep hypothermia is necessary to achieve adequate myoacardial protection during aortic cross-clamping. Anterograde cardioplegia combined with retrograde cardioplegia through the coronary sinus, and additional doses of cardioplegic solution not only through new saphenous vein grafts, but also through the arteriotomies prepared for

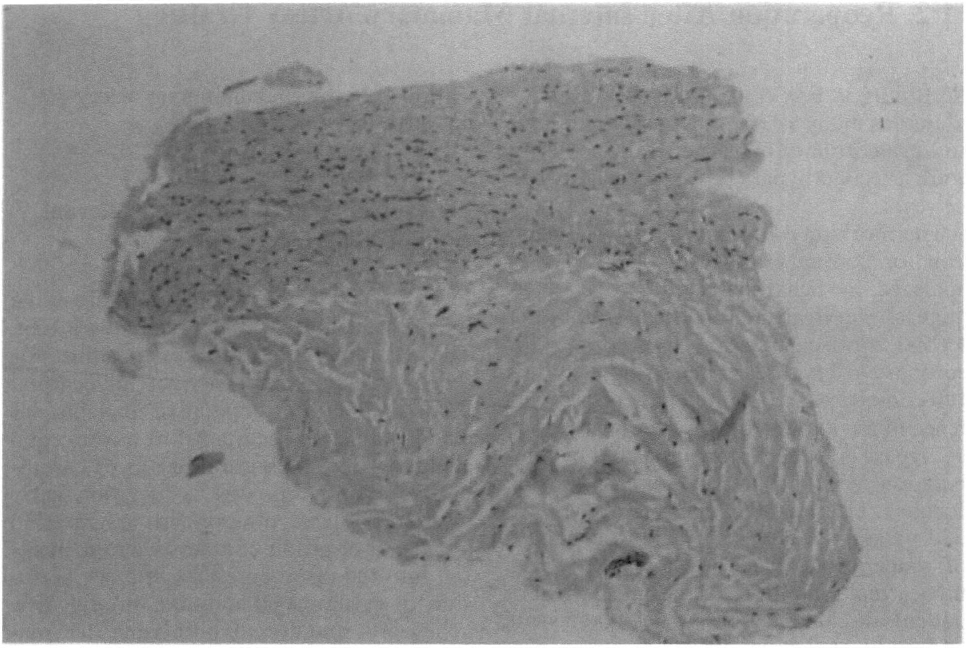

Fig. 125. Specimen of a left internal mammary artery revascularizing the left anterior descending coronary artery obtained 2 year after implantation at reoperation for stenosis distal of the anastomosis: moderate sclerosis. HE, ×20

Fig. 126. Specimen of a left internal mammary artery revascularizing the left anterior descending coronary artery obtained 6 months after implantation for stenosis of the internal mammary artery proximal to the anastomosis: significant periarterial reaction and moderate intimal hyperplasia. van Gieson

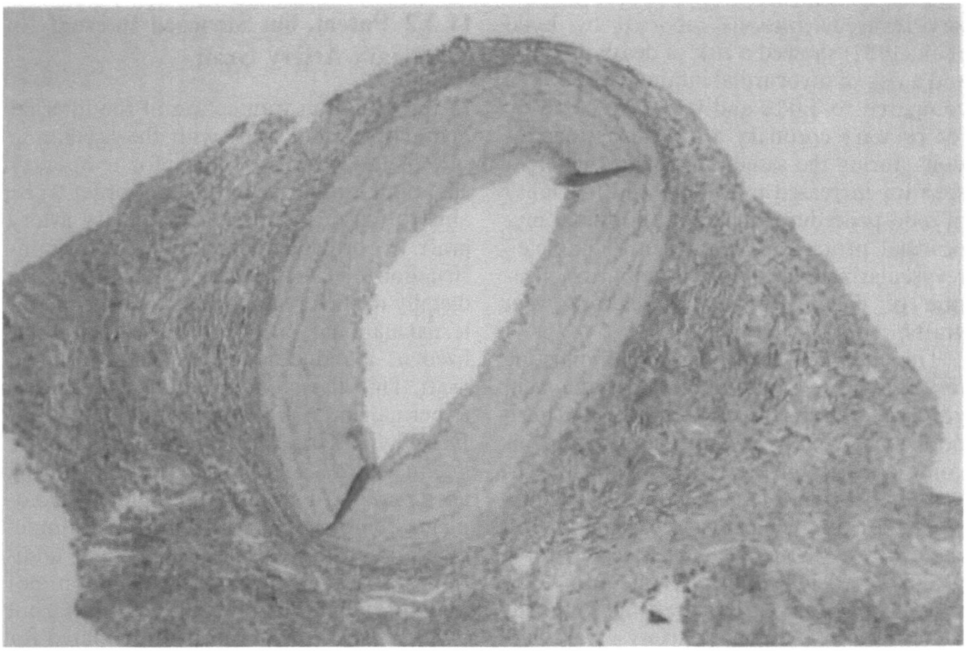

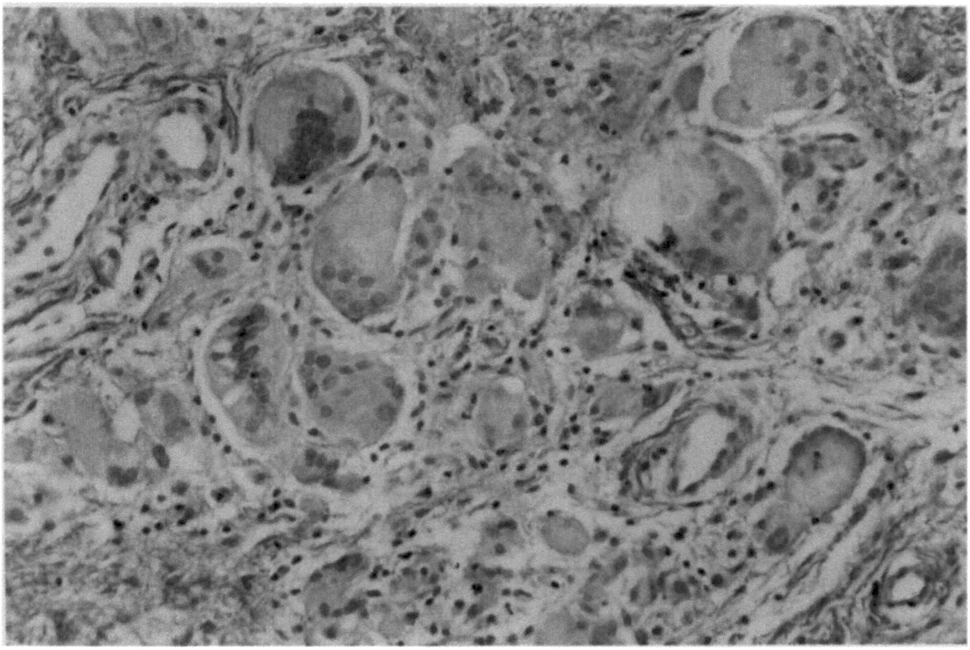

Fig. 127. Foreign body reaction 6 months after implantation of a left internal mammary artery onto the left anterior descending coronary artery: same specimen as Fig. 126. van Gieson

anastomoses with internal mammary artery grafts may help (see Sect. 7.3.3. for special cannulas etc).

A histologic sample of the distal end of an internal mammary artery obtained during a successful reoperation procedure performed 2 years after primary myocardial revascularization for progression of coronary artery disease and stenosis in the area of the internal mammary artery anastomosis is shown in Fig. 125. Another specimen from an internal mammary artery graft obtained at reoperation is shown in Fig. 126. Un uncommon foreign body reaction (Fig. 127) may have contributed to the moderate narrowing observed close to the distal anastomosis in this case.

11.2.3 Patent, not Stenosed Internal Mammary Artery Graft

In this situation, the transection of the internal mammary artery graft may be fatal if it occurs at an early stage of reoperation and use of a lateral thoracotomy approach for avoidance of patent anterior grafts at revisional coronary artery surgery has been suggested (Walker et al. 1986). If transection of the patent internal mammary artery graft occurs, a shunt may be useful for immediate reperfusion. Control of the patent internal mammary artery must, however be achieved to enable adequate cardioplegic arrest, to avoid rewarming of the myocardium and to avoid a suboptimal surgical field due to collateral blood flow. Again, deep hypothermia, anterograde and retrograde cardioplegia, and additional doses of cardioplegia through new vein grafts and arteriotomies as described above, may help to provide adequate myocardial protection during aortic cross-clamping.

The expected and observed difficulties at redo coronary artery revascularization after internal mammary artery grafting have led to the following recommendations during simple or expanded internal mammary artery grafting:

- Take down of the internal mammary arteries as pedicles to allow for dissection as a naked graft at later procedures,

- Right internal mammary artery grafts for revascularization of the left-sided coronary arteries should be routed through the transverse sinus,
- Protection of the internal mammary artery grafts from the sternal saw by lateral routing of the pedicles through the pericardium and adaptation of pleuropericardial flaps,
- Interposition of some tissue (e.g., thymus, pericardial and pleural fat)between the posterior sternal wall and the anterior surface of the heart and the great vessels,
- Closure, or adaptation of the pericardial sac whenever possible,
- Systematic use of the best grafting material available
- Complete revascularization at the primary procedure

12 Conclusion

Internal mammary artery bypass grafts implanted onto the left anterior descending coronary artery have shown superior long-term patency rates as compared to all other grafts and substitutes, resulting in improved long-term survival rates. The current trend to expanded internal mammary artery grafting using both internal mammary arteries is a logical step for further improvement of the results in coronary artery revascularization procedures.

However, one has to consider that internal mammary artery grafting is much more delicate than saphenous vein grafting and minor errors in technique or indication which may be harmless with the latter may lead to a disaster with the former. Therefore, good short-term results are necessary to achieve good long-term results; this fact has to be remembered when a patient is considered for expanded internal mammary artery grafting. Furthermore, the surgical population is changing: usually the patients have first been evaluated and rejected for percutaneous transluminal angioplasty and surgical revascularization is offered only in the group with more extensive coronary artery disease. This means that coronary bypass grafting is more needed and more complex in today's surgical patients.

Optimized coronary artery revascularization using both internal mammary arteries in combination with saphenous vein grafts is therefore recommended to take advantage of superior long-term patency rates of the internal mammary arteries and high initial flow rates of the saphenous vein grafts in the patient with so-called triple-vessel disease. As a matter of fact, resuscitation is extremely difficult if low cardiac output occurs for some reason and the myocardium is only supplied by the internal mammary arteries. Therefore, complex internal mammary artery grafting should not be used routinely if the entire myocardium or the major part of the left ventricle is at risk.

This strategy allows one to perform at least one internal mammary artery–coronary artery anastomosis in over 95% and multiple internal mammary artery–coronary artery anastomoses in over 50% of coronary artery revascularizations for an in-hospital mortality of less than 1% in scheduled cases of all ages. Further expansion of internal mammary artery grafting can be achieved by systematic multiple sequential grafting with bilateral in situ and/or free internal mammary arteries. However, as there are no reliable long-term results of this aggressive approach available today, the potential benefits have to be carefully balanced against the eventual drawbacks.

References

Aarnio P (1988) Free internal mammary artery graft as canine femoral artery substitute. Scand J Thor Cardiovasc Surg 1988, 22: 105–110

Aarnio P, Harjula ALJ, Viinikka L, Merikallio EM, Mattila SP (1988) Prostacyclin production in free versus native IMA grafts. Ann Thorac Surg 45: 390–392

Aarnio P, Järvinen A, Lehtola A, Merikallio E, Kivisaari L, Sariola H, Penttilä A (1989) The possibility of using celiac trunk branches as coronary artery bypass grafts. Scand J Thor Cardiovasc Surg 23: 165–168

Abe K, Main FB, Gerbode F (1966) Internal mammary-coronary artery anastomoses. A method utilizing Nakayama's instrument for small vessel anastomoses. J Thorac Cardiovasc Surg 51: 808–820

Adar R, Rubinstein Z, Hirshberg A (1988) Internal mammary artery coronary bypass and leg ischemia. J Vasc Surg 7: 820–821

Akins CW, Block PC, Palacios IF, Gold HK, Caroll DL, Grünkemeier GL (1989) Comparison of coronary artery bypass grafting and percutaneous transluminal coronary angioplasty as initial treatment strategies. Ann Thorac. Surg. 47: 507–516

Alderman EL, Fisher LD, Litwin P et al. (1983) Results of coronary artery surgery in patients with poor left ventricular function (CASS). Circulation 68: 785–795

Angelini GD, Christie MI, Bryan AJ, Lewis MJ (1989) Surgical preparation impairs release of endothelium-derived relaxing factor from human saphenous vein. Ann Thorac Surg 48: 417–20

Angell WW, Sywak A (1977) The saphenous vein versus internal mammary artery as a coronary bypass graft. Circulation 56 (suppl II): 11–22

Aris A, Borras X, Ramio J (1987) Patency of internal mammary artery grafts in no-flow situations. J Thorac Cardiovasc Surg 93: 62–64

Arnulf G (1948) La résection du plexus périaortique dans l'angine de poitrine. Arch Mal Coeur 42: 1191

Attum AA (1987) The use of the gastroepiploic artery for coronary artery bypass graft: another alternative. Texas Heart Institute Journal 14: 289–292

Barner HB (1973) The internal mammary artery as free graft. J Thorac Cardiovasc Surg 66: 219–221

Barner H.B. (1974a) Double internal mammary-coronary artery bypass. Arch Surg 109: 627–630

Barner HB (1974b) Internal mammary arteriography prior to coronary bypass. Chest 65: 703

Barner HB (1987) Flow through the internal mammary artery. J Thorac Cardiovasc Surg 93: 316–8

Barner HB, Mudd JG, Mark AL, Ahmad N, Dickens FD (1976) Patency of internal mammary-coronary grafts. Circulation 54 (Suppl 3): 70–73

Bartley TD, Bigelow JC, Page US (1972) Aortocoronary bypass grafting with multiple sequential anastomoses to a single vein. Arch Surg 105: 915

Bashour TT, Crew J, Kabbani SS, Ellertson D, Hanna ES, Cheng TO (1984) Symptomatic coronary and cerebral steal after internal mammary-coronary bypass. Am Heart J 108: 177–178

Bauer E, von Segesser L, Siebenmann R, Schneider K, Turina M (1988) Anomalies of internal mammary artery. Circulation 78 (Suppl 2): 477

Beavis RE, Mullany CJ, Cronin KD, et al (1988) An experimental in vivo study of the canine internal mammary artery and its response to vasoactive drugs. J Thorac Cardiovasc Surg 95: 1059–1066

Beck CS (1935) The development of a new blood supply to the heart by operation. Ann Surg 102: 801

Beck CS (1943) Principles underlying the operative approach to the treatment of myocardial ischemia. Ann Surg 118: 788–806

Beecher HK (1961) Surgery as placebo. A quantitative study of bias. JAMA 176: 1102–1107

Befeler B, Wells DE, Machado H, Thurer RJ, Castellanos A, Myerburg RJ (1975) Intercoronary steal syndrome resulting from aortocoronary bypass surgery. Am Heart J 89: 633–637

Bentall A, DeBono A (1968) A technique for complete replacement of the ascending aorta. Thorax 23: 338–339

Bertrand ME, Lablanche JM, Thieuleux F (1983) Rôle du spasme en pathologie coronarienne. Ann Chir Chir Thorac Cardio Vasc 37: 459–462

Bhayana JN, Gage AA, Takaro T (1980) Long term results of internal mammary artery implantation for coronary artery disease: a controlled trial by the participants of the Veterans Administration Coronary Bypass Surgery Cooperative Study Group. Ann Thorac Surg 29: 234–242

Bindslev L, Eklund J, Norlander O, Swedenborg J, Olsson P, et al (1987) Treatment of acute respiratory failure by extracorporeal carbon dioxide elimination performed with a surface heparinized artificial lung. Anesthesiology 67: 117–120

Björk VO, Ekeström S, Henze A, Ivert T, Landou C (1981a) Indications for the internal mammary artery graft. Scand J Thorac Cardiovasc Surg 15: 1–9

Björk VO, Ivert T, Landou C (1981b) Angiographic changes in internal mammary artery and saphenous vein grafts, two weeks, one year and five years after coronary bypass surgery. Scand J Thor Cardiovasc Surg 15: 23–30

Blesovsky A, Deal CW, Kerth WJ, Gerbode F (1967) Retrograde internal mammary artery implantation. J Thorac Cardiovasc Surg 53: 556–561

Bloomer WE., Bloor CM, Ellestad MH (1973) Functional studies of splenic and internal mammary artery implants in canine hearts. J Thorac Cardiovasc Surg 66: 222–234

Blumgart HL, Levine SA, Berlin DD (1933) Congestive heart failure and angina pectoris. The therapeutic effect of thyroidectomy on patients without clinical and pathological sign of thyroid toxicity. Arch Intern Med 51: 866–877

Boas EP (1926) The heart in thyroid disease. Med J Rec 124: 695–697

Boldt J, Kling D, von Bormann B, Züge M, Scheld H, Hempelmann G (1989) Blood conservation in cardiac operations. Cell separation versus hemofiltration. J Thorac Cardiovasc Surg 97: 832–840

Bourassa MG (1980) The role of bypass surgery in isolated left anterior descending artery stenosis or occlusion. Circulation 60: 875–876

Braunwald E (1983) Effects of coronary artery bypass grafting; Implications of the randomized coronary artery surgery study. N Engl J Med 309: 1181–1184

Braunwald E, Sonnenblick EH, Frommer PL et al. (1967) Paired electric stimulation of the heart. Physiologic observations and clinical implications. Adv Intern Med 13: 61–96

Brenot P, Mousseaux E, Relland J, Gaux JC (1988) Kinking of internal mammary grafts: report of two cases and surgical correction. Catheterization and Cardiovascular Diagnosis 14: 172–174

Brody WR, Kosek JC, Angell WW (1972) Changes in vein grafts following aortocoronary bypass induced by pressure and ischemia. J Thorac Cardiovasc Surg 64: 847

Brown AH (1977) Coronary steal by internal mammary graft with subclavian stenosis. J Thorac Cardiovasc Surg 73: 690–693

Bulkley BH, Hutchins GM (1977) Accelerated "atherosclerosis": a morphologic study of 97 saphenous vein coronary artery bypass grafts. Circulation 55: 163

Bundesamt für Statistik (1987) Statistisches Jahrbuch der Schweiz. Verlag Neue Zürcher Zeitung, Zürich

Bunzel B, Eckersberger F (1987) Veränderung der Lebensqualität nach aortokoronarem Bypass und Klappenersatz: ein Gradmesser des subjektiven Operationserfolges. Thorac Cardiovasc Surgeon 35: 242–247

Burgess GE, Cooper JR, Marino RJ, Peiler MJ, Mills NL Ochsner JL (1978) Pulmonary effect of pleurotomy during and after coronary artery bypass with internal mammary artery versus saphenous vein grafts. J Thorac Cardiovasc Surg 76: 230

Buxton AE, Goldberg S, Harken A, Hirshfeld J, Kastor JA (1981) Coronary artery spasm immediately after myocardial revascularization. Recognition and management. N Engl J Med 304: 1249–1253

Cabrol C, Pavie A, Mesnildrey P et al. (1986) Long term results with replacement of the ascending aorta and reimplantation of the coronary arteries. J Thorac Cardiovasc Surg 91: 17–25

Cachera JP, Loisance D, Gusmini D et al. (1982) Résultats à long terme des pontages aortocoronaires au cours des atteintes tri-tronculaires. Ann Chir: Chir Thorac Cardio-Vasc 36: 572–575

Cameron A, Kemp H, Shimomoura S, et al. (1979) Aortocoronary bypass surgery. A 7-year follow-up. Circulation 60 (Suppl) 1: 9–13

Cameron A, Kemp HG, Green GE (1986) Bypass surgery with the internal mammary artery graft: 15 year follow-up. Circulation 74 (suppl 3): 30–36

Cameron A, Kemp HG, Green GE (1988) Reoperation for coronary artery disease. 10 years follow-up. Circulation 78 (Suppl I): 158–162

Campeau L, Enjalbert M, Lesperance J, Vaislic C, Grondin CM, Bourassa MG (1983) Atherosclerosis and late closure of aortocoronary saphenous grafts. Sequential angiographic studies 2 weeks, 1 year, 5 to 7 years

and 10 to 12 years after surgery. Circulation 68 (Suppl 2):. 1
Carlson EB, Gilliam FR, Bashore TM (1988) Changes in epicardial coronary artery diameter following intracoronary papaverine in man. Catheterization and Cardiovascular Diagnosis 14: 150–153
Carpentier A, Guermonprez JL, Deloche A, Frechette C, DuBost C (1973) The aorto-to-coronary radial artery bypass graft. Ann Thorac Surg 16, 111–121
CASS Principal Investigators et al. (1983) Coronary artery surgery study (CASS): a randomized trial of coronary artery bypass surgery: survival data. Circulation 68: 939–950
Chaikhouni A, Crawford FA, Kochel PJ, Olanoff LS, Halushka PV (1986) Human internal mammary artery produces more prostacyclin than saphenous vein. J Thorac Cardiovasc Surg 92: 88–91
Chaitman BR, Davis KB, Dodge HT (1986) Should airline pilots be eligible to resume active flight status after coronary bypass surgery: a CASS registry study. J Am Coll Cardiol 8: 1318–1324
Chassignolle JF, Moreau JM, Mulsant P, et al. (1982) Valeur de l'anastomose mammaire interne-interventriculaire anterieure. Resultats sur une série consécutive de trois cent cinquante patients. Ann Chir Chir Thorac Cardio-Vasc 36: 601–604
Chaux A, Blanche C (1986) A new concept in sternal retraction: application for internal mammary artery dissection and valve replacement surgery. Ann Thorac Surg 42: 473–474
Chesebro JH, Frye RL (1983) Can myocardial function be improved by coronary bypass surgery. Cardiovascular Clinics 13: 221–238
Chesebro JH, Fuster V, Elreback LR, et al. (1984) Effect of dipyridamole and aspirin on late vein-graft patency after coronary bypass operations. N Engl J Med 1984 310: 209–214
Cheanvechai C, Garcia JM, Effler DB (1975) Internal mammary-coronary artery anastomosis. "No-touch" technique. Ann Thorac Surg 20: 709–712
Chiu CJ (1976) Why do radial artery grafts for aortocoronary bypass fail? A reappraisal Ann Thorac Surg 22: 520–523
Christian CB, Mack JW, Wetstein L (1985) Current status of coronary artery bypass grafting for coronary artery atherosclerosis. Surgical Clinics of North America 65: 509–526
Chuen-Neng L, Orszulak TA, Schaff HV, Kaye MP (1986) Flow capacity of the canine internal mammary artery. J Thorac Cardiovasc Surg 91, 405–410
Cobb LA, Thomas GI, Merendino KA, Bruce RA (1959) An evaluation of internal mammary artery ligation by a double blind technique. New Engl J Med 260: 1115
Cohen AJ, Ameika JA, Briggs RA, et al. (1988) Retrograde flow in the internal mammary artery. Ann Thorac Surg 45: 48–49
Cohn JN, Guiha NH, Broder MI, Constantinos JL (1974) Right ventricular infarction. Clinical and hemodynamic features. Am J Cardiol 33: 209–214
Coll-Mazzei J, Devolfe Ch, Adeleine P, et al. (1986) Aorto-coronary artery saphenous vein bypass surgery. A ten-year follow-up. J Cardiovasc Surg 27: 650–656
Collins JJ (1979) Direct myocardial revascularization (editorial comment). Am J Cardiol 43: 129–130
Collins JJ, Cohn LH, Sonnenblick EH, et al. (1973) Determinants of survival after coronary artery bypass surgery Circulation 48 (Suppl 3): 132–136
Conti CR, Pepine CJ, Curry RC (1979) Coronary artery spasm: an important mechanism in the pathophysiology of ischemic heart disease. Current Problems in Cardiology 4 (4): 1–70
Cooley DA (1983) Internal mammary-coronary artery bypass: experience with 1000 cases. Texas Heart Inst J 10: 223–224
Cooley DA, Wukasch DC, Bruno F et al.(1978) Direct myocardial revascularization with 9364 operations. Thorax 33: 411–417
Cosgrove DM, Loop FD (1985) Techniques to maximize mammary artery length. Ann Thorac Surg 40: 78–79
Cosgrove DM, Loop FD, Saunders CL Lytle BW, Kramer JR (1981) Should coronary arteries with less than fifty percent stenosis be bypassed? J Thorac Cardiovasc Surg 82: 520–530
Cosgrove DM, Loop FD, Lytle BW, et al. (1985a) Does mammary artery grafting increase surgical risk. Circulation 72 (Suppl 2): 170–174
Cosgrove DM, Loop FD, Lytle BW, et al. (1985b) Determinants of blood utilization during myocardial revascularization. Ann Thorac Surg 40: 380–384
Cosgrove DM, Loop FD, Lytle BW, et al. (1985c) Determinants of 10-year survival after primary myocardial revascularization. Ann Surg 202: 480–490
Cosgrove DM, Loop FD, Lytle BW, et al. (1986) Predictors of reoperation after myocardial revascularization. J Thorac Cardiovasc Surg 92: 811–821
Cosgrove DM, Lytle BW, Loop FD, et al. (1988) Does bilateral internal mammary artery grafting increase surgical risk. J Thorac Cardiovasc Surg 95: 850–856
Crosby IK, Craver JM (1975) The lesser saphenous vein. An alternative for coronary revascularization. Ann Thorac Surg 20: 703–705
Culliford AT, Cunningham JN, Zeff RH, Isom OW, Teiko P, Spencer FC (1976) Sternal and

costochrondral infections following open-heart surgery. A review of 2594 cases. J Thorac Cardiovasc Surg 72: 714–726
Cushing WJ, Magovern GJ, Olearchyk AS (1986) Internal mammary artery graft: retrospective report with 17 years' survival. J Thorac Cardiovasc Surg 92: 963–964
Curtis JJ, Stoney WS, Alford WC, Burrus GR, Thomas CS (1975) Intimal hyperplasia, a cause of radial artery aortocoronary bypass graft failure. Ann Thorax Surg 20: 628–635
Daly RC, McCarthy PM, Orszulak TA, Schaff HV, Edwards WD (1988) Histologic comparison of experimental coronary artery bypass grafts. Similarity of in situ and free internal mammary artery grafts. J Thorac Cardiovasc Surg 96: 19–29
Dardik H, Ibrahim IM, Sussman B et al. (1984) Biodegradation and aneurysm formation in umbilical vein grafts: Observations and a realistic strategy. Ann Surg 199: 61–68
Davies MJ, Thomas A (1984) Thrombosis and acute coronary artery lesions in sudden cardiac ischemic death. N Engl J Med 310: 1137–1140
De Servi S, Berzuini C, Ghio S, et al. (1988) Effects of surgical versus medical treatment on long-term prognosis in angina at rest: an observational non-randomized study of 400 patients. Eur Heart J 9: 513–519
Detre K (1986) Overview of coronary artery bypass graft surgery. Progress in Cardiovascular Diseases 28: 387–390
Di Summa M, Donegani E, Poletti GA (1988) Chylothorax after heart surgery. Minerva Cardioangiol (Ita) 36: 115–118
Dincer B, Barner HB (1983) The "occluded" internal mammary artery graft: Restoration of patency after apparent occlusion associated with progression of coronary disease. J Thorac Cardiovasc Surg 85: 318–320
Dobrin P, Canfield T, Moran J, Sullivan H, Pifarre R (1977) Coronary artery bypass. The physiological basis for differencies in flow with internal mammary artery and saphenous vein grafts. J Thorac Cardiovasc Surg 74: 445–454
Dorros G, Hale W, Deardorff W et al. (1981) Myocardial revascularization in a hemophiliac. Chest 79: 496
Edwards WS, Jones WB, Dear HD, Kerr AR (1970) Direct surgery for coronary artery disease. JAMA 211: 1182
Egloff L, Studer M, Rothlin M, Hess OM, Turina M, Senning A (1984) Koronare Reoperation – ja oder nein? Schweiz M Wochenschr 114: 1123–1126
Effler DB (1988) Vasilii I. Kolesov: Pioneer in coronary revascularization. J Thorac Cardiovasc Surg 96: 183
Effler DB, Favaloro RG, Groves LK, Loop FD (1971) The simple approach for direct coronary artery surgery. J Thorac Cardiovasc Surg 62: 503–510
Elayda MA, Hall RJ, Gray AG, Cooley DA (1984) Coronary revascularization in the elderly patient. J Am Coll Cardiol 3: 1398–1402
Ellestad MH (1971) Double-contrast angiography in human internal mammary implants. Ann Thorac Surg 12: 428–436
Elzinga WE, Skinner DB (1975) Hemodynamic characteristics of critical stenosis in canine coronary arteries. J Thorac Cardiovasc Surg 69: 217
Engelmann RM, Spencer FC, Boyd AD, Chandra R (1975) The significance of coronary arterial stenosis during cardiopulmonary bypass. J Thorac Cardiovasc Surg 70: 869–879
European Coronary Surgery Study Group (1980) Prospective randomized study of coronary artery bypass surgery in stable angina pectoris. Lancet 2: 491–495
European Coronary Surgery Study Group (1982) Long term results of prospective randomized study of coronary artery bypass surgery in stable angina pectoris. Lancet 11: 1173–1183
Faidutti B., von Segesser L. (1985) Secondary and late coronary artery bypass failure – actual technical indications. Helv Chir Acta 52: 397–405
Fauteaux M, Swenson O (1946) Pericoronary neurectomy in abolishing anginal pain in coronary disease. Arch Surg (Chicago) 53: 169
Favaloro R.G. (1968a) Double internal mammary artery implants. Operative technique. J Thorac Cardiovasc Surg 55: 457–465
Favaloro R.G. (1968b) Saphenous vein autograft replacement of severe segmental coronary artery occlusion - operative technique. Ann Thorac Surg 5: 334–339
Favaloro R.G. (1979) Direct myocardial revascularization: a ten year journey. Myths and Realities. Am J Cardiol 43: 109–129
Ferdinande PG, Beets G, Michels A, Lesaffre E, Lauwers P (1988) Pulmonary function tests after different techniques for coronary artery bypass surgery. Saphenous vein versus single versus double internal mammary artery grafts. Intensive Care Med 14: 623–627
Ferguson BT, Muhlbaier LH, Salai DL, Wechsler AS (1988) Coronary bypass gafting after failed elective and failed emergent percutaneous angioplasty. J Thorac Cardiovasc Surg 95: 761–762
Finci L, Meier B, Divernois J, Steffenino G, Melchior JP, von Segesser L, et al. (1987a) Traitement invasif de l'angor instable. Inf Cardio 11: 203–208
Finci L, von Segesser L, Meier B, et al. (1987b) Comparison of multivessel coronary angio-

plasty with surgical revascularization with both internal mammary arteries. Circulation 76 (Suppl 5): 1–6

Fiore AC, Naunheim KS, Kaiser GC, Willman VL, McBride LR, et al (1989) Coronary sinus versus aortic root perfusion with blood cardioplegia in elective myocardial revascularization. Ann Thorac Surg 47: 684–688

Fisk RL, Brooks CH, Callaghan JC, Dvorkin J (1976) Experience with the radial artery graft for coronary artery bypass. Ann Thorac Surg 21: 513–518

Fledge JB (1987) Pericardial incision for internal mammary artery coronary bypass. Ann Thorac Surg 44: 424

Flemma RJ, Johnson WD, Lepley D (1971) Triple aorto-coronary vein bypass as treatment for coronary insufficiency. Arch Surg 103: 82

Flemma RJ, Singh HM, Tector AJ, Lepley D, Frazier BL (1975) Comparative hemodynamic properties of vein and mammary artery in coronary bypass operations. Ann Thorac Surg 20: 619–627

Florian A, Lamberti JJ, Cohn LH, Collins JJ (1975) Revascularization of the right coronary artery by retrograde perfusion of the mammary artery. J Thorac Cardiovasc Surg 70: 19–23

Folts JD, Gallagher KP, Kroncke GM, Rowe GG (1981) Myocardial revascularization of the canine circumflex coronary artery using retrograde internal mammary artery flow without cardiopulmonary bypass. Ann Thorac Surg 31: 21–27

Fox MH, Gruchow HW, Barboriak JJ, et al. (1987) Risk factors among patients undergoing repeat aorto-coronary bypass procedures. J Thorac cardiovasc Surg 93: 56–61

Francois-Frank CE (1899) Signification physiologique de la résection du sympathique dans la maladie de Basedow, l'épilepsie, l'idiotie et le glaucome. Bull Acad Med Paris 41: 565

Frazier BL, Flemma RJ, Tector AJ, Korns ME (1974) Atherosclerosis involving the internal mammary artery. Ann Thorac Surg 18: 305–307

Frey RR, Bruscke AVG, Vermeulen FEE (1984) Serial angiographic evaluation 1 year and 9 years after aorto-coronary bypas. A study of 55 patients chosen at random. J Thorac Cardiovasc Surg 87: 167–174

Fuchs JCA, Mitchener JS, Hager PO (1978) Postoperative changes in autologous vein grafts. Ann Surg 188: 1

Furchgott RF, Zawadzky JV (1980) The obligatory role of endothelial cells in the relaxation of arterial smooth muscle by acetylcholine. Nature 299: 373–376

Furuse A, Klopp EH, Brawley RK, Gott VL (1972) Hemodynamics of coronary artery bypass. Ann Thorac Surg 14: 282

Fuster V, Chesebro JH (1986) Role of platelets and platelet inhibitors in aortocoronary artery vein-graft disease. Circulation 73: 227–232

Galbut DL, Traad EA, Dorman MJ, De Witt PL, Larsen PB et al. (1985) Twelve year experience with bilateral internal mammary grafts. Ann Thorac Surg 40: 264–270

Garrett HE, Dennis EW, De Bakey ME (1973) Aortocoronary bypass with saphenous vein graft: Seven year follow-up. JAMA 223: 792

Garrey WE, Atkins JA (1933) Cardiac innervation: Experimental and clinical studies. Arch Surg (Chicago) 26: 765

Gaudiani VA, Buch WS, Chin AK, Ayres LJ, Fogarty TJ (1988) An improved technique for the internal mammary artery coronary bypass graft procedure. J Cardiac Surg 3: 467–473

Geha AS (1976) Crossed double internal mammary-to-coronary artery grafts. Arch Surg 111: 289–292

Geha AS, Krone RJ, Mc Cormick JR, Baue AE (1975) Selection of coronary bypass: anatomic, physiological and angiographic considerations of vein and mammary artery grafts. J Thorac Cardiovasc Surg 70: 414

Gelbfish J, Jacobowitz IJ, Rose DM, et al. (1986) Cryopreserved homologous saphenous vein: Early and late patency in coronary artery bypass. Surgical procedures. Ann Thorac Surg 42: 70–73

Gersh BJ, Kronmal RA, Schaff HV, et al. (1985) Comparison of coronary artery bypass surgery and medical therapy in patients 65 years of age or older. N Engl J Med 313: 217–224

Goebel N, Pfluger N, Speiser K, Turina M, Rothlin M (1983) Veränderungen an den Nativgefässen nach aortokoronarer Bypassoperation. Fortschr Röntgenstr 139: 595–602

Goiti JJ, Smith GH (1982) Coronary artery surgery using inverted internal mammary artery. Br Heart J 48: 81–82

Gold JP, Shemin RJ, Di Sesa VJ, Cohn LH, Collins JJ (1985) Multiple-vessel coronary revascularization with combined in-situ and free sequential internal mammary arteries. J Thorac Cardiovasc Surg 90: 301

Golding LA, Loop FD, Hollmann JL, et al. (1986) Early results of emergency surgery after coronary angioplasty. Circulation 74 (Suppl 3): 26–29

Gott VL, Whiffen JD, Datton RC (1963) Heparin bonding on colloidal graphite surfaces. Science 142: 1297–1298

Graeber GM 1985) Creatine Kinase (CK): its use in the evaluation of perioperative myocardial infarction. Surgical Clinics of North America 65: 539–551

Green GE (1971) Rate of blood flow from the internal mammary artery. Surgery 70: 809–813

Green GE (1979) Technique of internal mammary-coronary artery anastomosis. J Thorac Cardiovasc Surg 78: 455–459
Green GE (1987) Technical factors influencing IMA graft patency. Ann Thorac Surg 44: 104–105
Green GE (1988) Use of the internal mammary artery in myocardial revascularization. Ann Thorac Surg 45: 453–454
Green GE, Som ML, Wolff WI (1965) Experimental microvascular suture anastomosis. Circulation 33 (Suppl I): 199
Green GE, Stertzer SH, Reppert EH (1968) Coronary arterial bypass grafts. Ann Thorac Surg 5: 443–450
Green GE, Kemp HG, Alam SE, Pierson RN, Friedman MI, David I (1979) Coronary bypass surgery. Five-year follow-up of a consecutive series of 140 patients. J Thorac Cardiovasc Surg 77: 48–56
Green GE (1989) Invited letter concerning: Preparation of the internal mammary artery graft: Which ist the best method? J Thorac Cardiovasc Surg 98: 152–153
Grondin CM, Lepage G, Catonquay Y, Mure C, Grondin P (1970) Initial blood flow through the graft and early postoperative patency. Circulation 42 (Suppl 3): 106
Grondin CM, Lesperance J, Bourassa MG, Campeau L (1975) Coronary artery grafting with the saphenous vein or internal mammary artery. Comparison of late results in two consecutive series of patients. Ann Thorac Surg 20: 605–617
Grondin CM, Campeau L, Lesperance J, Enjalbert M, Bourassa MG (1984) Comparison of late changes in internal mammary artery and saphenous vein grafts in two consecutive series of patients 10 years after operation. Circulation 70 (Suppl 1): 208–212
Grondin CM (1984) Late results of coronary artery grafting: is there a flag on the field? J Thorac Cardiovasc Surg 87: 161–166
Grüntzig A, Myler R, Hanna E, Turina M (1977) Transluminal angioplasty of coronary artery stenoses. Circulation 84 (Suppl 1): 56–57
Grüntzig AR, Senning A, Siegenthaler W (1979) Nonoperative dilatation of coronary artery stenosis. N Engl J Med 301: 61–68
Hahn C (1983) 14 Ans d'expérience en chirurgie de révascularisation directe du myocarde. Chirurgie 109: 702–713
Hamburg M, Swenson J, Wakabayashy T, Samuelsson B (1974) Prostaglandin endoperoxides. Novel transformations of arachidonic acid in human platelets. Proc Natl Acad Sci USA 71: 3400
Hamby RJ, Aintablian A, Wisoff BG, Hartstein ML (1977) Comparative study of the postoperative flow in the saphenous vein and internal mammary artery bypass grafts. Am Heart J 93: 306–315
Hanna ES, Kabbani SS, Bashour TT, et al. (1983) Internal mammary coronary artery bypass surgery: experience with 1000 cases. Texas Heart Inst J 10: 131–135
Harjola PT, Valle M (1974) The importance of aortic arch or subclavian angiography before coronary reconstruction. Chest 66: 436–438
Harjola PT, Frick MH, Harjula A, Järvinen A, Meurala H, Valle M (1984) Sequential internal mammary artery grafts in coronary artery bypass surgery. Thorac Cardiovasc Surgeon 32: 288–292
Hartz RS, Smith JA, Green D (1988) Autotransfusion after cardiac operation. Assessment of hemostatic factors. J Thorac Cardiovasc Surg 96: 178–182
Hasson JE, Newton WD, Waltman AC, et al. (1986) Mural degeneration in the glutaraldehyde-tanned umbilical vein graft: incidence and implications. J Vasc Surg 4: 243–250
Hirose T, Yaghmai M, Vera CA (1969) Cineangiographic visualization technique of the implanted right gastroepiploic artery of the posterior myocardium. Vasc Surg 3 (2): 61
Hochberg MS, Gielchinsky I, Parsonnet V, Hussain SM, Mirsky E, Fisch D (1989) Coronary angioplasty versus coronary bypass. Three-year follow-up of a matched series of 250 patients. J Thorac Cardiovasc Surg 97: 496–503
Hoffmann RG, Blumlein SL, Anderson AJ, Barboriak JJ, Walker JA, Rimm AA (1980) The probability of surviving coronary bypass surgery. Five-year results from 1718 patients. JAMA 243: 1341–1344
Huddleston CB, Stoney WS, Alford WC, et al. (1986) Internal mammary artery grafts: technical factors influencing patency. Ann Thorac Surg 42: 543–549
Huttunen H, Huttunen K, Tuppurainen T, Soimakallio S, Suhonen M (1989) Reversed left internal mammary artery graft for coronary bypass. Evaluation of function with digital subtraction angiography and radionuclide imaging. Scand J Thorac Cardiovasc Surg 23: 13–18
Isom OW, Spencer FC, Glassmann E, et al. (1978) Does coronary bypass increase longevity? J Thorac Cardiovasc Surg 75: 28–37
Ivert T, Huttunen K, Landou C, Björk VO (1988) Angiographic studies of internal mammary artery grafts 11 years after coronary artery bypass grafting. J Thorac Cardiovasc Surg 86: 1–12
Jahnke EJ, Love JW (1976) Bypass of the right and circumflex coronary arteries with the internal mammary artery. J Thorac Cardiovasc Surg 71: 58–63
Jett GK, Arcidi JM, Dorsey LMA, Hatcher CR,

Guyton RA (1987) Vasoactive drugs effects on blood flow in internal mammary artery and saphenous vein graft. J Thorac Cardiovasc Surg 94: 2–11
Johns RA, Peach MJ, Flanagan T, Kron IL (1989) Probing the canine mammary artery damages endothelium and impairs vasodilatation resulting from prostacyclin and endothelium derived relaxing factor. J Thorac Cardiovasc Surg 97: 252–258
Johnson WD, Flemma RJ, Manley JC, Lepley D (1970) The physiological parameters of ventricular function as affected by direct coronary surgery. J Thorac Cardiovasc Surg 60: 483
Johnson AM, Kron IL, Watson DD, Gibson RS, Nolan SP (1986) Evaluation of postoperative flow reserve in internal mammary artery bypass grafts. J Thorac Cardiovasc Surg 92: 822–826
Jones M, Conkle DM, Ferrans VJ, et al. (1973) Lesions observed in arterial autogenous vein grafts. Light and electron microscopic evaluation. Circulation 48 (Suppl 3): 198–210
Jones JM, Ochsner JL, Mills NL, Hughes L (1978) The internal mammary bypass graft: a superior second coronary artery. J Thorac Cardiovasc Surg 75: 625
Jones JM, Ochsner JL, Mills NL, Hughes L (1980) Clinical comparison between patients with saphenous vein and internal mammary artery as coronary graft. J Thorac Cardiovasc Surg 80: 334–341
Jonnesco T. (1920) Traitement chirurgical de l'angine de poitrine par la résection du sympathique cervico-thoracique. Bull Acad Med Paris 84: 93
Jonsson K, Karlsson S (1985) Angiography of the internal mammary artery. Acta radiologica 26: 113–120
Jülke M, von Segesser L, Schneider J, Turina M, Heitz PU (1989) Ausmass der Arteriosklerose der Arteria mammaria interna und der Koronararterien bei Männern im Alter von 45 bis 75 Jahren. Eine Autopsie Studie. Schweiz M Wochenschr 119: 1219–1223
Kabbani SS, Hanna ES, Bashour TT, Crew JR, Ellertson DG (1983) Sequential internal mammary-coronary artery bypass. J Thorac Cardiovasc Surg 86: 697–702
Kamath ML, Matysik LS, Schmidt DH, Smith LL (1985) Sequential internal mammary artery grafts. Expanded utilization of an ideal conduit. J Thorac Cardiovasc Surg 89: 163–169
Kanter KR, Barner HB (1987) Improved technique for the proximal anastomosis with free internal mammary artery grafts. Ann Thorac Surg 44: 556–557
Kay EB, Naraghipour H, Beg RA, DeManey M, Tambe A, Zimmermann HA (1974) Internal mammary artery bypass graft - long-term patency rate and follow-up. Ann Thorac Surg 18: 269–279
Kay HJ, Korns ME, Flemma RJ, Tector AJ, Lepley D (1976) Atherosclerosis of the internal mammary artery. Ann Thorac Surg 21: 504–507
Kennedy JW, Kaiser GC, Fisher LD, et al. (1980) Multivariate discriminant analysis of the clinical and angiographic predictors of operative mortality from the collaborative study in coronary artery surgery (CASS). J Thorac Cardiovasc Surg 80: 876–887
Keon WJ, Akyurekli Y, Bedard P et al. (1979) Coronary endarteriectomy: an adjunct to coronary artery bypass grafting. Surgery 86: 859–867
Killip T (1988) Twenty years of coronary bypass surgery. New Engl J Med 319: 366–368
Kirklin JW, Barrat-Boyes BG (1986) Cardiac Surgery. Wiley Inc, New York, pp 207–277
Knapp WS, Douglas JS, Craver JM, et al. (1981) Efficacy of coronary bypass grafting in elderly patients with coronary artery disease. Am J Cardiol 47: 923–930
Kolesov VI (1967) Mammary artery-coronary artery anastomosis as method of treatment for angina pectoris. J Thorac Cardiovasc Surg 54: 535–44
Kolesov VI (1982) Remote results of mammary-coronary anastomosis. Vestn Khir 1: 49–53
Kolesov VI, Potashov LV (1965) Operations on the coronary arteries. Exp Chir Anaesth 10: 3–8
Kuttler H, Hauenstein KH, Kameda T, Wenz W, Schlosser V (1988) Significance of early angiographic follow-up after internal thoracic artery anastomosis in coronary surgery. Thorac Cardiovasc Surgeon 36: 96–99
Landymore RW, Chapman DM (1987) Anatomical studies to support the expanded use of the internal mammary artery graft for myocardial revascularization. Ann Thorac Surg 44: 4–6
Largiadèr J (1985) Below knee reconstructions with the human umbilical veins - three years results. Thorac cardiovasc Surgeon 33: 377–381
Largiadèr J, Peter M (1987) A surgical strategy for femoro-crural reconstruction. Eur J Vasc Surg 1: 205–212
Lee CN, Orszulak TA, Schaff HV, Kaye MP (1986) Flow capacity of the canine internal mammary artery. J Thorac Cardiovasc Surg 91: 405–410
Lefrak EA (1987) The internal mammary artery bypass: praise versus practice. Texas Heart Inst J 14: 139–143
Lehmann KH, von Segesser L, Müller-Glauser W, Siebenmann R, Schneider K et al. (1989) Superior results with internal mammary-coro-

nary artery anastomoses due to better preservation of the endothelium. Thorac Cardiovasc Surgeon 37: 187–189
Lehtola A, Verkkala K, Järvinen A (1989) Is electrocautery safe for internal mammary artery mobilization? A study using scanning electron microscopy (SEM). Thorac Cardiovasc Surgeon 37: 55–57
Leitmann IM, Paull DE, Barie PS, Isom OW, Shires GT (1987) Intra-abdominal complications of cardiopulmonary bypass operations. Surg Gynecol Obstet 165: 251–254
Lindenau KF, Bohm J, Scholz B, et al. (1976) Morphologische und angiographische Untersuchungen der A. mammaria interna bei Koronarsklerose. Z Exper Chirurg 9: 155–160
Lioupis A (1988) Early mortality after isolated coronary artery bypass graft operations. Inaugural Dissertation, Zürich University Hosital
Livi U, Campalani G, Ross DN (1986) Distal internal mammary artery (IMA) with retrograde flow for coronary artery grafting. Thorac Cardiovasc Surgeon 34: 204–206
Longmire WP, Cannon JA, Kattus AA (1958) Direct vision coronary endarterectomy for angina pectoris. N Engl J Med 259: 993
Loop FD (1979) Technique for performance of internal mammary artery-coronary artery anastomosis. J Thorac Cardiovasc Surg 78: 460–463
Loop FD, Spampinato N, Siegel W, et al. (1973) Internal mammary artery grafts without optical assistance. Circulation 48 (Suppl 3): 162–167
Loop FD, Carabajal NR, Taylor PC, Irarrazaval MJ (1976) Internal mammary artery bypass graft in reoperative myocardial revascularization. Am J Cardiol 37: 890–895
Loop FD, Irarrazaval MJ, Bredee JJ, Siegel W, Taylor PC, Sheldon WC (1977) Internal mammary artery graft for ischemic heart disease. Effect of revascularization on clinical status and survival. Am J Cardiol 39: 516–522
Loop FD, Cosgrove DM, Lytle BW, et al. (1979) An 11 year evolution of coronary arterial surgery (1967–1978). Ann Surg 190: 444–455
Loop FD, Sheldon WC, Lytle BW, Cosgrove DM, Proudfit WL (1981) The efficacy of coronary artery surgery. Am Heart J 101: 86–96
Loop FD, Lytle BW, Cosgrove DM, et al. (1986a) Influence of the internal mammary artery graft on 10-year survival and other cardiac events. N Engl J Med 314: 2–6
Loop FD, Lytle BW, Cosgrove DM, Golding LAR, Taylor PC, Stewart RW (1986b) Free (aorto-coronary) internal mammary artery graft. Late results. J Thorac Cardiovasc Surg 92: 827–831
Love JW, Jahnke EJ, McFadden RB, et al. (1980) Myocardial revascularization in patients with chronic renal failure. J Thorac Cardiovasc Surg 79: 625–627
Lüscher TF, Diederich D, Siebenmann R, Lehmann K, Stultz P, von Segesser L, et al. (1988) Difference between endothelium-dependent relaxation in arterial and in venous coronary artery bypass grafts. N Engl J Med 319: 462–467
Lye CR, String ST, Wylie EJ, Stoney RJ (1975) Aortorenal arterial autografts. Arch Surg 1975, 110: 1321–1326
Lytle BW, Loop FD, Thurer RL, Groves LK, Taylor PC, Cosgrove DM (1980) Isolated left anterior descending coronary atherosclerosis: long-term comparison of internal mammary artery and venous autografts. Circulation 61: 869–874
Lytle BW, Loop FD, Cosgrove DM, et al. (1983) Long-term (5–12 years) sequential studies of internal mammary artery and saphenous vein coronary bypass garfts. Circulation 68 (Suppl 3): 114
Lytle BW, Cosgrove DM, Loop FD, et al. (1986) Perioperative risk of bilateral internal mammary artery grafting: analysis of 500 cases from 1971 to 1984. Circulation 74 (Suppl 3): 37–41
Lytle BW, Loop FD, Cosgrove DM, et al. (1987) Fifteen hundred coronary reoperations. Results and determinants of early and late survival. J Thorac cardiovasc Surg 93: 847–859
Maher TD, Glenn JF, Magovern GJ (1982) Internal mammary arteriovenous fistula after sternotomy. Arch Surg 117: 1100–1101
Malone JM, Kischer CW, Moore WS (1981) Changes in venous endothelial fibrinolytic activity and histology with in vitro venous distension and arterial implantation. Am J Surg 142: 178
Mandl F (1925) Die Anwendungsbreite der paravertebralen Injektion bei der Angina pectoris. Klin Wchnschr 4 2356
Marshall WG, Miller EC, Kouchoukos NT (1988) The coronary-subclavian steal sysndrom: report of a case and recommendations for prevention and management. Ann Thorac Surg 46: 93–96
Martinez MJ, Garcia-Rinaldi R, Traad EA (1988) Minimizing internal mammary artery anastomotic tension. Ann Thorac Surg 46: 712
Mayou R, Bryant B (1987) Quality of life after coronary artery surgery. Q J Med New Series 62 (239): 239–248
McCallister BD, Richmond DR, Saltups A, Hallermann FJ, Wallace RB, Frye RL (1970) Left ventricular hemodynamics before and 1 year after internal mammary artery implantation in patients with coronary artery disease and angina pectoris. Circulation 52: 471–477
McConn RL, Hagen PO, Fuchs JCA (1980) As-

pirin and dipyridamole decrease intimal hyperplasia in experimental vein grafts. Ann Surg 191: 238
McCormick JR, Kaneko M, Baue AE, Geha AS (1975) Blood flow and vasoactive drug effects in internal mammary and venous bypass grafts. Circulation 52 (Suppl 1): 72–80
McEachern CG, Manning GW, Hall GE (1940) Sudden occlusion of coronary arteries following removal of cardiosensory pathways: experimental study. Arch Intern Med 65: 661–670
McGeachie J, Campbell P, Prendergast F (1981) Vein to artery grafts. A quantitative study of revascularization by vaso vasorum and its relationship to intimal hyperplasia. Ann Surg 194: 100
Meier B (1988) Restenosis after coronary angioplasty: review of the literature. Eur Heart J 9 (Suppl C): 1–6
Meier B, Rutishauser W (1985) Transluminal coronary angioplasty - state of the art 1984. Acta Med Scand 701 (Suppl): 142–147
Meier B, Chaves V, von Segesser L, Faidutti B, Rutishauser W (1985) Vocational rehabilitation after coronary angioplasty and coronary bypass surgery. In: Walter PJ (ed) Return to work after coronary bypass surgery. Psychosocial and economic aspects. Springer Berlin Heidelberg New York, pp 171–176
Mestres CA, Rives A, Igual A, Vehi C, Murta M (1986) Atherosclerosis of the internal mammary artery. Histopathological analysis and implications of its results in coronary artery bypass graft surgery. Thorac Cardiovasc Surgeon 34: 356–358
Mills NL, Bringaze WL (1989) Preparation of the internal mammary artery graft: Which is the best method ? J Thorac Cardiovasc Surg 98: 73–79
Mills NL, Everson CT (1989a) Right gastrepiploic artery: A third arterial conduit for coronary artery bypass. Ann Thorac Surg 47: 706–11
Mills NL, Everson CT (1989b) Technical considerations for use of the gastroepiploic artery for coronary artery surgery. J Cardiac Surg 4: 1–9
Mitchel BF, Adam M, Lambert CJ, Sunger S, Shiekh S (1970) Ascending aorto-to-coronary artery saphenous vein bypass grafts. J Thorac Cardivasc Surg 54: 535
Molina JE, Carr M, Yarnoz MD (1978) Coronary bypass with Gore-Tex graft. J Thorac Cardiovasc Surg 75: 769–771
Moncada S, Vane JR (1980) Prostacyclin in the cardiovascular system. Adv Prostaglandin Thromboxane Leukotriene Res 6: 43–60
Mullen DC, Lepley D, Flemma RJ (1977) Cronary artery surgery without global ischemia. Ann Thorac Surg 24: 90–91
Müller-Glauser W, Lehmann KH, Bittmann P, Bay U, Dittes P, von Segesser L, Turina M (1988) A compliant small-diameter vascular prosthesis lined with functional venous endothelial cells. Trans Am Soc Artif Intern Organs 34: 528–531
Mullerworth MH, Daniel FJ, Lie JT (1975) The fate of internal mammary arterial implants and bypass conduits for myocardial revascularization. J Thorac Cardiovasc Surg 70: 89–99
Murray G, Porcheron R, Hilario J, Roschlau W (1954) Anastomosis of a systemic artery to the coronary. Can Med Assoc J 71: 594
Myers WO, Schaff HV, Fisher LD, et al. (1988) Time to first new myocardial infarction in patients with severe angina and three-vessel disease comparing medical and early surgical therapy: a CASS registry study of survival. J Thorac Cardiovasc Surg 95: 382–389
Myles EL (1988) Carbodissection of the internal thoracic artery pedicle. Ann Thorac Surg 46: 470–471
Nakatsuka M, Colquhoun A, Gehr L (1989) Right ventricular function and high-frequency positive-pressure ventilation during coronary artery bypass grafting. Ann Thorac Surg 48: 263–266
National Heart, Lung and Blood Institute (1981) Coronary Artery Surgery Study. Principal investigations of CASS and their associates. Circulation 63: 1–143
Nemes A, Sotonyi P, Balogh A, Nagy SJ (1977) Verwendung der A. mammaria interna zur myokardialen Revaskularisation. Acta Chir Acad Sci Hung 18: 123–128
Neutze JM, White HD (1987) What contribution has cardiac surgery made to the decline in mortality from coronary heart disease. Br Med J 294: 405–409
New York Heart Association (1964) Diseases of the heart and blood vessels - nomenclature and criteria for diagnosis. Little Brown, Boston
Ni Y, von Segesser LK, Turina M (1990) Futility of pericardiectomy for post-radiation constricting pericarditis? Ann Thorac Surg 49: 445–448
Nkongho A, Luber JM, Bell-Thomson J, Green GE (1984) Sternotomy infection after harvesting of the internal mammary artery. J Thorac Cardiovasc Surg 88: 788–789
Nojiri C, Noishiki Y, Koyanagi H (1987) Aortocoronary bypass grafting with heparinized vascular grafts in dogs. J Thorac Cardiovasc Surg 93: 867–877
Oakley CM (1986) Surgery and prognosis in coronary heart disease. Q J Med New Series 60 (231): 637–641
Oakley CM (1987) Is there life after coronary ar-

tery surgery. Q J Med New Series 62 (239): 181–182
Okies JE, Page US, Bigelow JC, Krause AH, Salomon NW (1984) The left internal mammary artery: the graft of choice. Circulation 70 (Suppl 1): 213–221
Olearchyk AS (1986) History of coronary artery bypass grafting. J Ukr Med Assoc North Am 33: 3–8
Olearchyk AS (1988) Vasilii I Kolesov - A pioneer of coronary revascularization by internal mammary-coronary artery grafting. J Thorac Cardiovasc Surg 96: 13–18
Olearchyk AS, Magovern GJ (1986) Internal mammary artery grafting: Clinical results, patency rates and long term survival in 833 patients. J Thorac Cardiovasc Surg 92: 1082–1087
Olson CG, Dunton RF, Maggs PR, Lahey SJ (1988) Review of coronary-subclavian steal following internal mammary artery-coronary artery bypass surgery. Ann Thorac Surg 46: 675–678
Passamini E, Davis KB, Gillespie MJ, Killip T, CASS Principal Investigators et al. (1985) A randomized trial of coronary artery bypass surgery: survival of patients with low ejection fraction. N Engl J Med 312: 1665–1671
Payen D, Bousseau D, Laborde F, Beloucif S, Menu P, Compos A, Echter E, Piwnica A (1986) Comparison of perioperative and postoperative phasic blood flow in aortocoronary venous bypass grafts by means of pulsed Doppler echocardiography with implantable microprobes. Circulation 74 (Suppl 3): 61–67
Pelias AJ, Del Rossi AJ (1985) A case of postoperative internal mammary steal. J Thorac Carduiovasc Surg 90: 794–795
Perrenoud JJ, Hauser H, Bopp P, Hahn C, Rutihauser W (1981) Valeur de la tomoradiométrie transverse dans le contrôle de la perméabilite des ponts aorto-coronaires par rapport à la coronarographie. Arch Mal Coeur 74: 41–48
Pharma Information (1988) Das Gesundheitswesen in der Schweiz. Leistungen Kosten Preise. Basel
Pichard AD, Ambrose J, Mindich B, et al. (1980) Coronary artery spasm and perioperative cardiac arrest. J Thorac Cardiovasc Surg 80: 249–245
Pidgeon J, Treasure T, Brooks N, Cattel M, Balcon R (1984) Correlation of angiographic and surgical findings in distal coronary branches. Br Heart J 51: 125–129
Prieto I, Basile F (1982) L'angine instable: traitment chirurgical à l'Hôtel-Dieu de Montreal. Union Med Canada 111: 1063–1066
Pryor DB, Harrell FE, Rankin JS, et al. (1987) The changing survival benefits of coronary revascularization over time. Circulation 76 (suppl V): 13–21
Puig LB, Ciongolli W, Cividanes GVL et al. (1990) Inferior epigastric artery as free graft for myocardial revascularization. J Thorac Cardiovasc Surg 99: 251–255
Pym J, Brister SJ, Brown PM, Charrette EPJ, Gutelius JR (1987) Technique and results of gastro-epiploic to coronary bypass. J Cardiovasc Surg 28: 3
Rainer WG, Sadler TR, Liggett MS (1973) Internal mammary arteriography prior to coronary bypass surgery. Chest 64: 523–524
Rankin JS, Newmann GE, Bashore TM, et al. (1986) Clinical and angiographic assessment of complex mammary artery bypass grafting. J Thorac Cardiovasc Surg 92: 832–846
Reul GJ (1985) Present status of the internal mammary artery as a coronary artery bypass conduit at the Texas Heart Institute. Texas Heart Inst J 12: 211–219
Rivera R, Duran E, Ajuria M (1988) Expanded use of the right and left internal mammary arteries for myocardial revascularization. Thorac Cardiovasc Surgeon 36: 194–197
Robicsek F, Sanger PW, Daugherty HK, Galluci V (1967) Origin of the anterior interventricular (descending) coronary artery and vein from the left mammary vessels. J Thorac Cardiovasc Surg 53: 602–604
Robinson PS, Coltart J, Jenkins BS et al. (1978) Coronary artery surgery: indications and recent experience. Postgrad Med J 54: 649–657
Ross R, Glomset J, Karya B, Harker L (1974) A platelet dependent serum factor that stimulates the proliferation of arterial smooth muscle cells in vitro. Proc Natl Acad Sci 71: 1207
Royston D, Taylor KM, Bidstrup BP, Sapsford RN (1987) Effect of Aprotinin on need for blood transfusion after repeat open heart surgery. Lancet, December 5: 1289–1291
Rutishauser W, Simon H, Stucky JP, Schad N, Noseda G, Wellauer J (1967) Evaluation of roentgen cinedensitometry for flow measurements in models and in the intact circulation. Circulation 36: 951
Rutishauser W, Bussmann W, Noseda G, Meier W, Wellauer J (1970) Blood flow measurement through single coronary arteries by roentgen densitometry. Part I. A comparison of flow measured by a radiological technique applicable in the intact organism and by electomagnetic flowmeter. Am Heart J 109: 12
Sarabu M, McKlung J, Fass A, Reed G (1987) Early postoperative spasm in left internal mammary artery bypass graft. Ann Thorac Surg 44: 199–200
Sauvage LR, Wu H, Kowalsky TE, et al. (1986) Healing basis and surgical techniques for complete revascularization of the left ventricle using only the internal mammary arteries. Ann Thorac Surg 42: 449–465

Schaff HV, Orszulak TA, Gersh BJ, et al. (1983) The morbidity and mortality of reoperation for coronary artery disease and analysis of late results with use of actuarial estimate of event-free interval. J Thorac Cardiovasc Surg 85: 508–515

Schimert G, Vidne BA, Lee AB (1975) Free internal mammary artery graft. An improved surgical technique. Ann Thorac Surg 19: 474–477

Schmidt DH, Blau F, Hellman C, Grzelak L, Johnson WD (1980) Isoproterenol-induced flow responses in mammary and vein bypass grafts. J Thorac Cardiovasc Surg 80: 319–326

Schulman ML, Bradhey MR (1982) Late results and angiographic evaluation of arm veins as long bypass conduits. Surgery 92: 1032

Selzer A (1983) Aortocoronary bypass in asymptomatic or mildly symptomatic coronary patients. Am J Cardiol 51: 1043–1042

Senning A (1961) Strip grafting in coronary arteries: report of a case. J Thorac Cardiovasc Surg 41: 542

Sergeant P, Wouters L, Dekeyser L, Flameng W, Suy R (1986) Is the outcome of coronary artery bypass graft surgery predictable in patients with severe ventricular function impairment? J Cardiovasc Surg 27: 618–621

Sewell WH (1974) Improved coronary vein graft patency rates with side to side anastomosis. Ann Thorac Surg 17: 538

Shaw PJ, Bates D, Cartlidge NEF et al. (1987) Long-term intellectual dysfunction following coronary artery bypass graft surgery: a six month follow-up study. Q J Med 1987, New Series 62 (239): 259–268

Shine TSJ, Scarborough CJ, Barnhorst DA, Finck SJ (1988) High-frequency ventilation during dissection of the internal mammary artery. Ann Thorac Surg 46: 256

Showstack JA, Rosenfeld KE, Garnick DW, Luft HS, Schaffarzick RW, Fowles J (1987) Association of volume with outcome of coronary artery bypass graft surgery - scheduled versus nonscheduled operations. JAMA 257/6: 785–789

Siegel W, Loop FD (1976) Comparison of internal mammary artery and saphenous vein bypass grafts for myocardial revascularization: exercise test and angiographic correlations. Circulation 54 (Suppl 3): 1–3

Singh RN (1980) Internal mammary arteriography. A new catheter technique by right brachial approach. Cathet Cardiovasc Diagn 6: 439–449

Singh RN, Magovern GJ (1982) Internal mammary graft: improved flow resulting from correction of steal phenomenon. J Thorac Cardiovasc Surg 84: 146–148

Singh RN, Sosa JA (1981) Internal mammary-coronary artery anastomosis. Influence of side branches on surgical results. J Thorac Cardiovasc Surg 82: 909–914

Singh RN, Sosa JA (1984) Internal mammary artery: a "live" conduit for coronary bypass. J Thorac Cardiovasc Surg 87: 936–938

Singh RN, Varat MA (1982) Coronary artery spasm occurring late after vein graft surgery. Cathet Cardiovasc Diagn 8: 617–622

Singh RN, Sosa JA, Green GE (1983) Internal mammary artery versus saphenous vein graft. Comparative performance in patients with combined revascularization. Br Heart J 5O: 48–58

Singh RN, Beg RA, Kay EB (1986) Physiological adaptability: the secret of success of the internal mammary artery grafts. Ann Thorac Surg 41: 247–50

Singh RN, Beg RA, Kay EB (1987) Flow capacity of the human internal mammary artery. J Thorac Cardiovasc Surg 97: 316

Skidgel RA, Printz MP (1978) PGI_2 production by rat blood vessels. Diminished prostacyclin formation in veins compared to arteries. Prostaglandins 16: 1–15

Smith HC, Frye RL, Piehler JM (1983) Does coronary bypass surgery have a favorable influence on the quality of life. Cardiovasc Clinics 13: 253–264

Sones FM, Shirey EK (1962) Cine coronary arteriography. Mod Concepts Cardiovasc Dis 31: 735

Speiser K, Rothlin M, Turina M (1983) Comparison between internal mammary artery implantation and aorto-coronary vein bypass grafting in coronary artery disease with significant left anterior descending stenosis. Thorac Cardiovasc Surgeon 31: 54–57

Spencer FC (1983) Surgical management of coronary artery disease. In: Sabiston DC, Spencer FC, (eds) Gibbon's surgery of the chest, W. B. Saunders, Philadelphia, Vol II, pp 1424–1451

Spencer FC (1986) The internal mammary artery: the ideal coronary bypass graft. N Engl J Med 314: 50–51

Spencer FC, Yong NK, Prachubrioh K (1964) Internal-mammary-coronary anastomoses performed during cardiopulmonary bypass. Thorac Cardiovasc Surg 5: 292

Spray TL, Roberst WC (1977) Changes in saphenous veins used as aortocoronary bypass grafts. Am Heart J 94: 500

Starr DS, Moore JP (1989) Localized pericardial flap to prevent tension on left internal mammary artery grafts. Ann Thorac Surg 47: 623–624

Steffenino G, Meier B, Bopp L, Finci L, von Segesser L, et al. (1985) Non-selective intra-arterial digital subtraction angiography for the

assessement of coronary artery bypass grafts. Int J Cardiac Imaging 1: 209–215
Steffenino G., Meier B., Finci L., von Segesser L., Velebit V. (1986) Percutaneous transluminal angioplasty of right and left internal mammary artery grafts. Chest 90: 849–851
Stoney RJ, Wylie EJ (1970) Arterial autografts. Surgery 67: 18–25
Subramanian VA, Hernandez Y, Tack-Goldman K, Grabowski EF, Weksler BB (1986) Prostacyclin production by internal mammary artery as a factor in coronary artery bypass grafts. Surgery 100: 376–381
Suma H, Takeuchi A, Hirota Y (1989) Myocardial revascularization with combined arterial grafts utilizing the internal mammary and the gastroepiploic artery. Ann Thorac Surg 47: 712–715
Suzuki A, Kay EB, Hardy JD (1973) Direct anastomosis of the bilateral internal mammary artery to the distal coronary,without a magnifier, for severe diffuse coronary atherosclerosis. Circulation 48 (Suppl 3): 190–197
Szilagyi DE, Elliot JP, Hageman JH, Smith RF, Dall-Olmo CA (1973) Biologic fate of autogenous vein implants as arterial substitutes. Ann Surg 178: 232
Takaro T, Hultgren HN, Kopton MJ, Dete KM (1976) The VA cooperative randomized study for coronary arterial occlusive disease. II. Subgroup with significant left main lesions. Circulation 54 (Suppl III): 107–117
Takaro T, Bhayana J, Dean D (1985) Veterans administration cooperative study of medical versus surgical treatment for stable angina – progress report. Prog Cardiovasc Dis 28: 213–218
Tanimoto Y, Matsuda Y, Masuda T et al. (1990) Multiple free (aorto-coronary) gastroepiploic artery grafting. Ann Thorac Surg 49: 479–480
Tartini R, Steinbrunn W, Kappenberger L, Goebel N, Turina M (1985) Anomalous origin of the left thyrocervical trunk as a cause of residual pain after myocardial revascularization with internal mammary artery. Ann Thorac Surg 40: 302–304
Tector AJ (1986) Fifteen years' experience with the internal mammary artery graft. Ann Thorac Surg 42 (Suppl): S22–S27
Tector AJ, Schmahl TM, Canino VR (1983) The internal mammary artery graft: the best choice for bypass of the diseased left anterior descending coronary artery. Circulation 68 (Suppl 2): 214–217
Tector AJ, Schmahl TM, Canino VR, Kallies JR,-Sanfilippo D (1984) The role of the sequential internal mammary artery graft in coronary surgery. Circulation 70 (Suppl 1): 222–225
Tector AJ, Schmahl TM, Canino VR (1986) Expanding the use of the internal mammary artery to improve patency in coronary artery bypass grafting. J Thorac Cardiovasc Surg 91: 9–16
Thom TJ, Kannel WB (1981) Downward trend in cardiovascular mortality. Annu Rev Med 32: 427
Tice DA, Zerbino VR, Isom OW, Cunningham JN, Engelman RM (1976) Coronary artery bypass with freeze-preserved saphenous vein allografts. J Thorac Cardiovasc Surg 71: 378–382
Tobler HG, Edwards JE (1988) Frequency and location of atherosclerotic plaques in the ascending aorta. J Thorac Cardiovasc Surg 96: 304–306
Todd EP, Earle GF, Jaggers R, Sekela M (1987) Pericardial flap to minimize internal mammary artery anastomotic tension. Ann Thorac Surg 44: 665
Turina M (1983) Instabile Angina pectoris: Chirurgische Behandlung. Verh Dtsch Ges Herz Kreislaufforschg 49: 35–40
Turina M (1987) Ändert sich die Indikation zur aorto-koronaren Bypassoperation? Internist 28: 747–750
Turina M and von Segesser L (1989) Coronary bypass grafting for acute, myocardial infarction after angioplasty and thrombolysis. Current Opinion in Cardiology 4: 789–792
Tyras DH, Barner HB (1977) Coronary-subclavian steal. Arch Surg 112: 1125–1127
Tyras DH, Barner HB, Kaiser GC, Codd JE, Pennington DG, Willman VL (1980) Bypass grafts to the left anterior descending coronary artery. Saphenous vein versus internal mammary artery. J Thorac Cardiovasc Surg 80: 327–333
Ulliot DJ (1980) Current controversies in the conduct of the coronary bypass operation. Ann Thorac Surg 30: 192–203
Underwood SR (1988) Magnetic resonance imaging of the cardiovascular system. Curr Med Lit Cardiovasc Med 7: 95–101
Urschel HC, Morales AR (1967) Posterior myocardial revascularization by retrograde internal mammary artery implantation. Surgery 61: 59–73
Valentine RJ, Fry RE, Wheelan KR, Fisher DF, Clagett GP (1987) Coronary-subclavian steal from reversed flow in an internal mammary artery used for coronary bypass. Am J Cardiol 59: 719–720
Vander Salm TJ, Chowdhary S, Okike ON, Pezzella AT, Pasque MK (1989) Internal mammary artery grafts: The shortest route to the coronary arteries. Ann Thorac Surg 47: 421–427
Varnauskas E, European Coronary Surgery Study Group (1988). Twelve-year follow-up of survival in the randomized European coro-

nary surgery study. N Engl J Med 319: 332–337
Velican C., Velican D. (1976) Intimal thickening in developing coronary arteries and its relevance to atherosclerotic involvement. Atherosclerosis 23: 345
Verkkala K, Järvinen A, Keto P, Virtanen K, Lehtola A, Pellinen T (1989) Right gastroepiploic artery as coronary bypass graft. Ann Thorac Surg 47: 716–719
Veterans Administration Coronary Artery Bypass Surgery Cooperative Study Group (1984) Eleven-year survival in the Veterans Administration randomized trial of coronary bypass surgery for stable angina. N Engl J Med 311: 1333–1339
Vineberg AM (1946) Development of anastomosis between coronary vessels and transplanted internal mammary artery. Can Med Assoc J 55: 117–119
Vineberg AM, Miller G (1951) Internal mammary coronary anastomosis in the surgical treatment of coronary artery insufficiency. Can Med Assoc J 64: 204
Vogel JHK, McFadden RB, Spence R, Jahnke EJ, Love JW (1978) Quantitative assessment of myocardial performance and graft patency following coronary bypass with the internal mammary artery. J Thorac Cardiovasc Surg 75: 487
von Segesser L (1987) Determination of significant differencies in performance of the Bentley BOS-CM 40 hollow fiber membrane oxygenator and the Polystan VT5000 venotherm bubble oxygenator. Perfusion 2: 289–295
von Segesser L, Faidutti B (1984) Pontages femoro-jambiers. A propos de 106 pontages consecutifs. J Chir (Paris) 121: 401–409
von Segesser L, Faidutti B (1988) Infected sternotomy following cardiac surgery. Reconstr Surg Traumat 20: 94–100
von Segesser L, Turina M (1987) Surgical revascularization after balloon angioplasty. Curr Opinion Cardiol 2: 1023–1026
von Segesser L, Turina M (1989) Cardiopulmonary bypass without systemic heparinization: performance of heparin-coated oxygenators in comparison with classic membrane and bubble oxygenators. J Thorac Cardiovasc Surg 98: 386–396
von Segesser L, Turina M (1990) Künstliche Ventrikel als Brücke zur Herztransplantation. Therapeutische Umschau 47: 129–132
von Segesser L, Leuenberger A, Faidutti B (1985) Multiple internal mammary-coronary artery anastomoses. Eur Heart J 6: 129
von Segesser L, Leuenberger A, Neidhart P, Faidutti B (1986a) Revascularisations coronariennes par anastomoses mammaires multiples en comparaison avec les greffons veineux classiques. Schweiz Med Wochenschr 116: 1621–1623
von Segesser L, Cox J, Faidutti B (1986b) Equine pericardial xenograft in orthotopic position: early results. Thorac Cardiovasc Surgeon 34: 35–38
von Segesser L, Abdesselam N, Schneider PA, Faidutti B (1986c) La revascularisation des artères viscérales (rénales et digestives) chez le jeune adulte: évolution de la tactique chirurgicale. Helv Chir Acta 53: 95–99
von Segesser L, Jornod N, Faidutti B (1987a) Repeat sternotomy after reconstruction of the pericardial sac with glutaraldehyde-preserved equine pericardium. J Thorac Cardiovasc Surg 93: 616–619
von Segesser L, Simonet F, Meier B, Finci L, Faidutti B (1987b) Inadequate flow after internal mammary-coronary artery anastomoses. Thorac cardiovasc Surgeon 35: 352–354
von Segesser L, Meier B, Finci L, et al. (1987c) La chirurgie des lesions anévrysmales des artères coronaires. Helv Chir Acta 54: 233–237
von Segesser L, Leskosek B, Redha F, Hänseler R, Tornic M, Turina M (1988) Performance characteristics of a disposable ventricle assist device. Thorac Cardiovasc Surgeon 36: 146–150
von Segesser L, Lehmann K, Turina M (1989a) Deleterious effects of shock in internal mammary artery anastomoses. Ann Thorac Surg 47: 575–579
von Segesser L, Schneider K, Siebenmann R, Turina M (1989b) Blutersatz bei Herztransplantation. (in Beitr Infusionsther 24: 159–164)
von Segesser L, Lehmann K, Turina M (1989c) Retrograde internal mammary-coronary artery anastomoses. Thorac Cardiovasc Surgeon 37: 143–146
von Segesser L, Lachat M, Leskosek B, Garcia E, Turina M (1990a) An open membrane oxygenator system with the safety of a closed system. (in press)
von Segesser L, Garcia E, Turina M (1990b) A convertible cardiopulmonary bypass system for optimized hemofiltration. J Extra-Corp Technol 22: 8
von Segesser L, Weiss B, Garcia E, Gallino A, Turina M (1990c) Reduced blood loss and transfusion requirements with low systemic heparinization: preliminary clinical results in coronary artery revascularization. Eur J Cardiothorac Surg: in submission
Wakabayashi A, Connolly JE (1968) Comparative flow studies of myocardial revascularization grafts. J Thorac Cardiovasc Surg 56: 633–642
Walker WS, Sang CTM (1986) Avoidance of

patent anterior grafts at revisional coronary artery surgery: use of a lateral thoracotomy approach. Thorax 41: 692–695
Waller BF, Roberts WC (1980) Amount of narrowing by atherosclerotic plaque in 44 nonbypassed and 52 bypassed major epicardial coronary arteries in 32 necropsy patients who died within 1 month of aortocoronary bypass grafting. Am J Cardiol 46: 956–962
White JC, Sweet WH (1955) Pain: Its Mechanisms and Neurosurgical Control. Charles C. Thomas, Springfield, Ill. USA
Wilcox P, Baile EM, Hards J, Müller NL, Dunn L, et al. (1988) Phrenic nerve function and its relationship to atelectasis after coronary artery bypass surgery. Chest 93: 693–698
Williams CD (1989) Retrocaval route for coronary bypass grafting. J Cardiac Surg 4: 104–108
William-Olsson G., Otoya E., Ekeström S. (1968) The initial flow in a myocardial vessel implant in the dog. Scand J Cardiovasc Surg 2: 200–202
William-Olsson G (1971) Pressure in the intramyocardially implanted internal mammary arteries in dogs in relation to aortic pressure and depth of implant. Scand J Thorac Cardiovasc Surg 5: 243–245
Wolinsky H (1980) A proposal linking clearance of circulating lipoproteins to tissue metabolic activity as a basis for understanding atherogenesis. Circ Res 47: 301
Woodring JH, Royer JM, Todd EP (1985) Upper rib fractures following median sternotomy. Ann Thorac Surg 39: 355–357
Yokoyama M, Sakakibara S (1972) Blood flow measurements in internal mammary artery implanted into the myocardium. Ann Thorac Surg 13: 155–162
Zakhour BJ, Drucker MH, Franco AA (1988) Chylothorax as a complication of aortocoronary bypass. Two case reports and a review of the literature. Scand J Thor Cardiovasc Surg 22: 93–95
Zeff RH, Kongtahworn C, Iannone LA, et al. (1988) Internal mammary artery versus saphenous vein graft to the left anterior descending coronary artery: Prospective randomized study with 10-year follow-up. Ann Thorac Surg 45: 533–536

Subject Index

Suppliers of Material

Abiomed,
Cherry Hill Drive,
Danvers, Massachusetts 01923,
Unitd States

AB Stille-Werner,
Förmansvägen 2,
P.O. Box 43051,
S-100 72 Stockholm,
Sweden

Atrium Medical Corporation,
17 Clinton Drive,
Hollis, New Hampshire 03049,
United States

Baxter Healthcare Corpororation,
Bentley Laboratories Inc and Edwards
CVS Division,
17502 Armstrong Avenue,
Irvine, California 92714–5686,
United States

Bio-Vascular Inc,
2670 Patton Road,
Saint Paul, Minnesota 55113,
United States

Codman & Shurtleff Inc,
Randolph, Massachusetts 02368,
United States

C. R. Bard Inc,
1425 South Village Way,
Santa Ana, California 92705,
United States

Datascope Corp,
P.O. Box 5,
Paramus, New Jersey 07653–005,
United States

Davis & Geck, Cyanamid International,
Wayne, New Jersey 07470,
United States

Delacroix–Chevalier,
13 Avenue de la République,
75011 Paris,
France

Dideco S.p.A.,
Via Galilei,
41037 Mirandola,
Italy

dlp Inc,
620 Watson S.W.,

Grand Rapids, Michigan 49504
United States

Gambro Dialisatoren KG,
7450 Hechingen,
Federal Republic of Germany

Gaymar Industries Inc,
Orchard Park,
New York 14127
United States

Gebrüder Martin,
Postfach 60,
7200 Tuttlingen,
Federal Republic of Germany

Haemonetics Corporation,
400 Wood Road,
Braintree, Massachusetts 02148,
United States

HyCult bv,
P.O. Box 595,
5400 AN Uden,
The Netherlands

Johnson & Johnson Corporation,
1 Johnson & Johnson Plaza
New Brunswick, New Jersey 08933
United States

Lucius & Baer GmBH,
Sperlingstrasse 1,
8192 Geretsried 1,
Federal Republic of Germany

Medinvent SA,
1000 Lausanne,
Switzerland

Millar Instruments Inc,
6001 Gulf Freeway,
Houston, Texas 77023
United States

Omnitract,
Minnesota Scientific Inc,
3839 Chandler Drive N. E.,
Minneapolis, Minnesota 55421
United States

Pilling,
420 Delaware Drive,
Fort Washington, Pennsylvania 19034,
United States

Sarns Inc/3M,
Ann Arbor, Michigan 48103,
United States

Scanlan International Inc,
One Scanlan Plaza,
Saint Paul, Minnesota 55107,
United States

Schneider-Shiley,
Schärenmoosstrasse 115,
8052 Zürich,
Switzerland

Sechrist Industries Inc,
Medical Products Division,
2820 Gretta Lane,
Anaheim, California 92806,
United States

Sharpoint Inc,
2850 Windmill Road,
Reading, Pennsyslvania 19608,
United States

Snowdon, Pencer Inc,
Tucker, Georgia
United States

Stöckert Instrumente GmbH,
Osterwaldstrasse 10,
8000 München 40,
Federal Republic of Germany

Titanium Manufacture Belge de Gembloux S.A.,
Rue Albert 9,
5800 Gembloux,
Belgium

T. Koros Surgical Instruments Corporation
Moorpark, California 93021
United States

Ulrich AG,
Bahnhofstrasse 11,
9000 St Gallen,
Switzerland

Valleylab Inc Surgical Products,
5920 Longbow Drive,
P.O. Box 9015,
Boulder, Colorado 80301,
United States

MIX
Papier aus verantwortungsvollen Quellen
Paper from responsible sources
FSC® C105338

If you have any concerns about our products,
you can contact us on
ProductSafety@springernature.com

In case Publisher is established outside the EU,
the EU authorized representative is:
Springer Nature Customer Service Center GmbH
Europaplatz 3, 69115 Heidelberg, Germany

Printed by Libri Plureos GmbH
in Hamburg, Germany